ॐ

ARNAVH YOGA

7 Steps 7 Minutes

TOTAL CONTROL 7ASPECTS

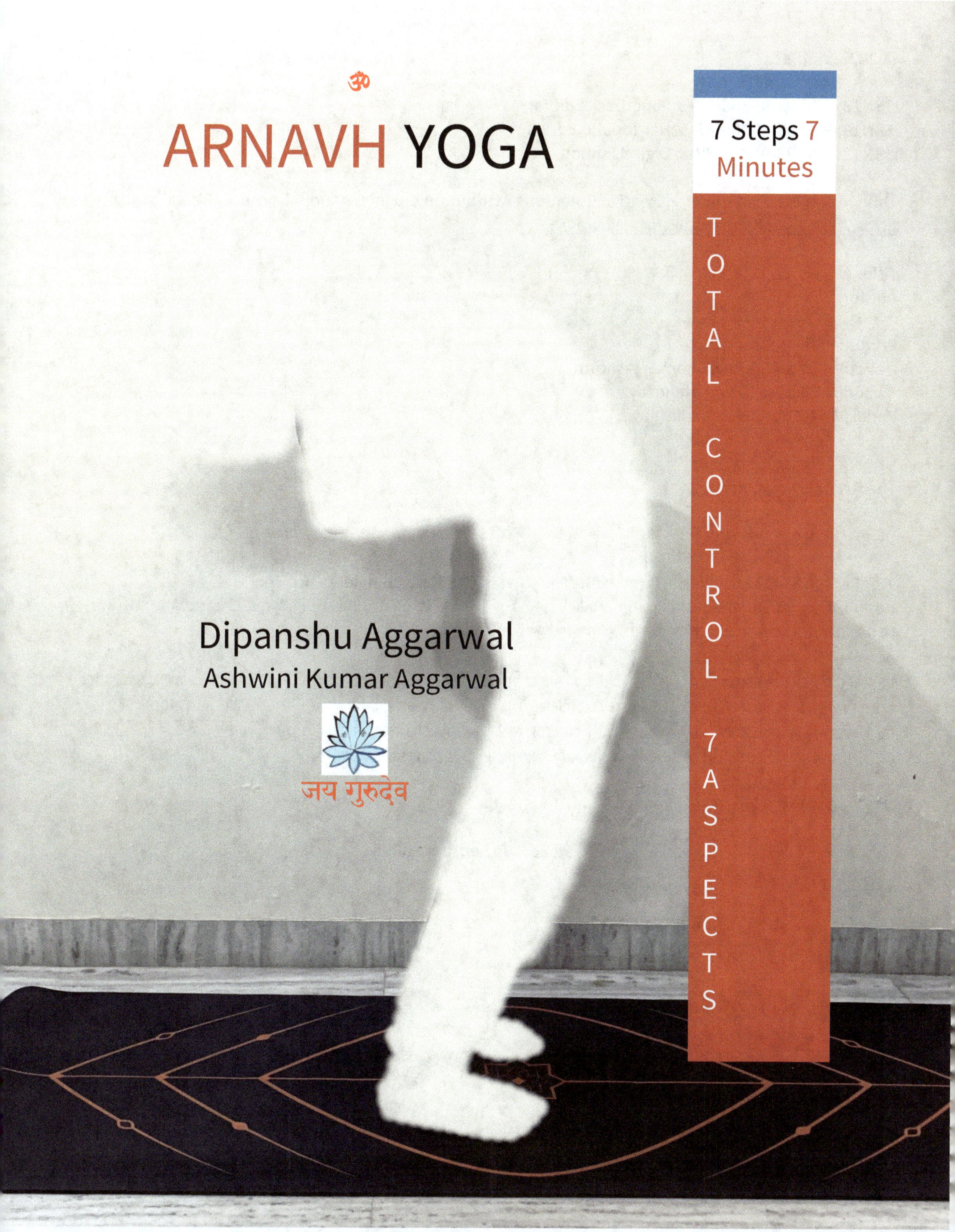

Dipanshu Aggarwal

Ashwini Kumar Aggarwal

जय गुरुदेव

ISBN13: 978-93-95766-37-1 Paperback Edition
ISBN13: 978-93-95766-42-5 Hardbound Edition
ISBN13: 978-93-95766-38-8 Digital Edition

Title: **Arnavh Yoga**
Author: **Ashwini Kumar Aggarwal, Dipanshu Aggarwal**

Printed and Published by
Devotees of Sri Sri Ravi Shankar Ashram
34 Sunny Enclave, Devigarh Road,
Patiala 147001, Punjab, India

https://advaita56.in/
The Art of Living Centre

https://www.artofliving.org/

18th February 2023, Maha Shivaratri Rudra Puja at Helios Club, Sunview Enclave.
Basant Ritu, Phalguna Masa, Krishna Paksha, Shani Trayodashi Tithi, Pradosh Vrat, Uttarayana, Uttara Ashadha upari Shravana Nakshatra, Sarvartha Siddhi Yoga.

On this day on 3102 BC Epoch of Kali Yuga, 1678 AD John Bunyan's book Pilgrim's Progress published, 1879 French sculptor Frederic-Auguste Bartholdi awarded a patent for designing Statue of Liberty, 1885 Mark Twain's novel Adventures of Huckleberry Finn published, 1977 Space Shuttle Enterprise's maiden flight atop a Boeing 747 aircraft, 2023 Today 150000+ people from 60 nations participate in Mahashivratri celebrations at Bangalore Ashram.

Vikram Samvat 2079 Nala, Saka Era 1944 Shubhakrit

1st Edition February 2023

जय गुरुदेव

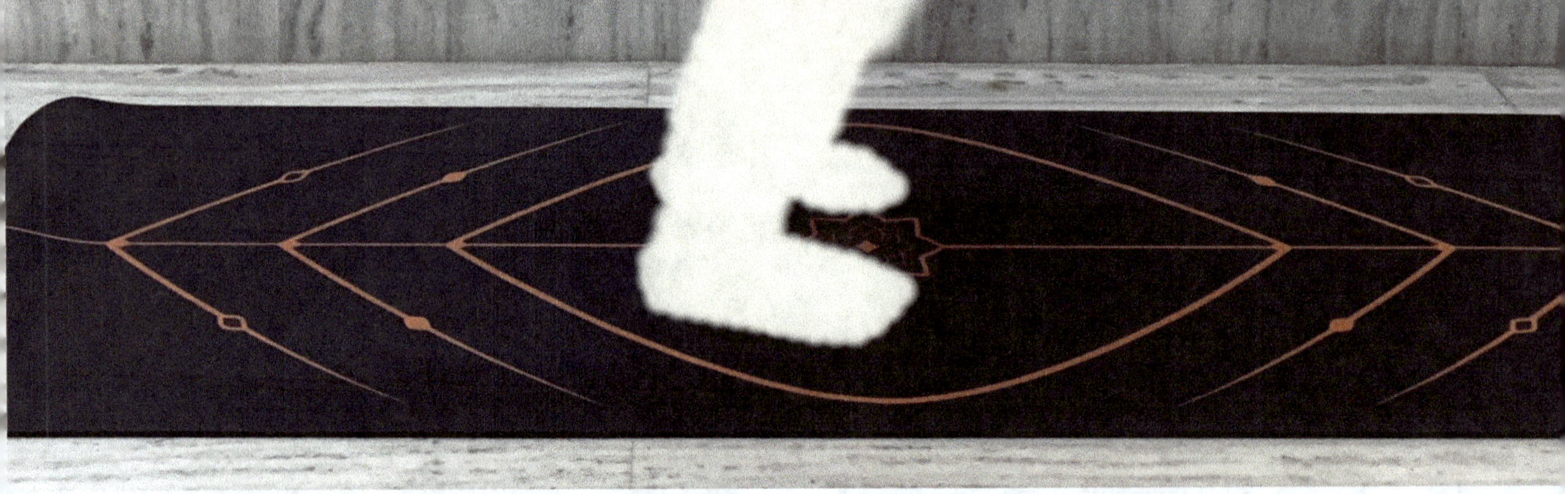

Dedication

Sri Sri Ravi Shankar

who revealed to us the **Sudarshan Kriya**
5 March 1981 Shimoga
https://www.youtube.com/watch?v=zn9AsGvmUyA

an offering at thy lotus feet

Editorial and Content Design Creation Team

Dipanshu, Richa, Radhika, Pavani, Himika, Laxmi & Kritansha, Hema

Acknowledgements

Adapted from our widely used title "Yoga Science and Practice" iSBN 9788194619802

Front Cover Image Credits

Dipanshu on the Yoga mat. Photo dated 16 May 2021.

Inspiration from contemporary Yogis

Krishan Verma https://shudham.org/

Kashi Bhaiya https://twitter.com/dkashikar

Jagjit Singh https://sunviewenclave.com/
Kamlesh Barwal https://twitter.com/kamleshbarwal
Dr Shilajeet Banerjee https://profiles.stanford.edu/shilajeet-banerjee
Dr Surekha Bhanot https://www.researchgate.net/profile/Surekha_Bhanot
Dr Mandeep Singh https://scholar.google.co.in/citations?user=s9vTtMMAAAAJ&hl=en
Laura Gnecco https://www.instagram.com/lauragneccoflow/?hl=en

7 Steps 7 Minutes

TOTAL CONTROL 7 ASPECTS

Blessing

It's not important that you can barely touch your toes or strike advanced poses or recite the Patanjali Yoga Sutras by heart.

What's important is the length of your smile, no matter what's happening in the world.

The total prana is represented by one syllable OM. Before birth, we were part of that sound and after death we will merge with that sound

the SOUND of the Spirit.

Sri Sri Ravi Shankar

Contents

BLESSING 4

PRAYER 6

WHAT IS YOGA 7

ETYMOLOGY 7

PROPS DEEPEN THE YOGA EXPERIENCE 9

YOGA MAT & WATER BOTTLE 9

YOGACHARYA'S GRACE 11

0 BREAK NOTIONS, CONCEPTS LET GO 12

1 ADVANCED POSTURES 12

LOTUS POSE - PADMĀSANA 13
BACK STRETCH - PASCHIMOTTANĀSANA 17
WHEEL POSE - CHAKRĀSANA 21
TREE - VRIKSHĀSANA 25
BUTTERFLY – TITLI ĀSANA 29
HEADSTAND - SHIRSĀSANA 33
RELAXATION POSES 36
CORPSE POSE - SHAVĀSANA 37
CROCODILE - MAKARĀSANA 40
PRONE VISHNU 43
FAMILY INVOLVING CHILDREN 47

TO SUMMARIZE

4 GOOD BATH 51

7 PRANAYAMA 52

UJJAYI BREATH 52
BHASTRIKĀ 53
NADI SHODHANA 56
PRATYAHARA INWARD TURN 59
DHARANA CONCENTRATION 59

2 MEDITATION DHYANA 60

IMPORTANCE OF GUIDED MEDITATION 61
HARI OM MEDITATION 61
PANCAKOSHA MEDITATION 61
SAMADHI TRANSCENDENTAL STATE 62

3 WALKING 63

5 OUTDOOR SPORTS 64

6 HAVAN 65

REGULAR HABITS 66

WATCH YOUR TONGUE 66
PRAYER CHANTING AND SINGING 66
DIET 67
MARMA, MERU CHIKITSA, CRANIOSACRAL THERAPY REFLEXOLOGY 67
PANCHAKARMA 67
EYE CARE & TOOTH CARE 68
MUDRA AND BANDHA 69
YOGA IS A FAMILY THING 69

ASANA HANDOUT 71

WALL SUPPORT 72

TRADITIONAL TEXTS 73

YOGA VASISTHA 73
BHAGAVAD GITA 74
PATANJALI YOGA SUTRAS 75
THIRUMOOLAR MANTHIRAM 76
HATHA YOGA PRADIPIKA 77
GHERANDA SAMHITA 78

SURYA NAMASKARS FOR HEALTH, EFFICIENCY & LONGEVITY 79
SUGGESTED READING 79

EPILOGUE **80**

Prayer

ॐ भद्रं कर्णेभिः शृणुयाम देवाः । भद्रं पश्ये माक्षभिर् यजत्राः ।
स्थिरैरङ्गैस् तुष्टुवा(गुं)सस्तनूभिः । व्यशेम देवहितं यदायुः ॥
स्वस्ति न इन्द्रो वृद्धश्रवाः । स्वस्ति नः पूषा विश्ववेदाः ।
स्वस्ति नस्तार्क्ष्यो अरिष्टनेमिः । स्वस्ति नो बृहस्पतिर्दधातु ॥
ॐ शान्तिः शान्तिः शान्तिः ॥

oṃ bhadraṃ karṇebhiḥ śṛṇuyāma devāḥ I bhadraṃ paśye mākṣabhir yajatrāḥ I sthirairaṅgais tuṣṭuvā(guṃ)sastanūbhiḥ I vyaśema devahitaṃ yadāyuḥ II svasti na indro vṛddhaśravāḥ I svasti naḥ pūṣā viśvavedāḥ I svasti nastārkṣyo ariṣṭanemiḥ I svasti no bṛhaspatirdadhātu II
oṃ śāntiḥ śāntiḥ śāntiḥ II

O Divine Glow!
May our ears listen to the sacred and the auspicious.
May our eyes see the propitious as we join to partake of wisdom.
May our limbs be firm and body attuned to long endurance.

May our senses function with full alertness and
May the emotion of contentment be fulsome.
May our good thoughts form a discus to shield us and
May our education give us a shining personality.
Peace in our heart, in our body, and in our environs.

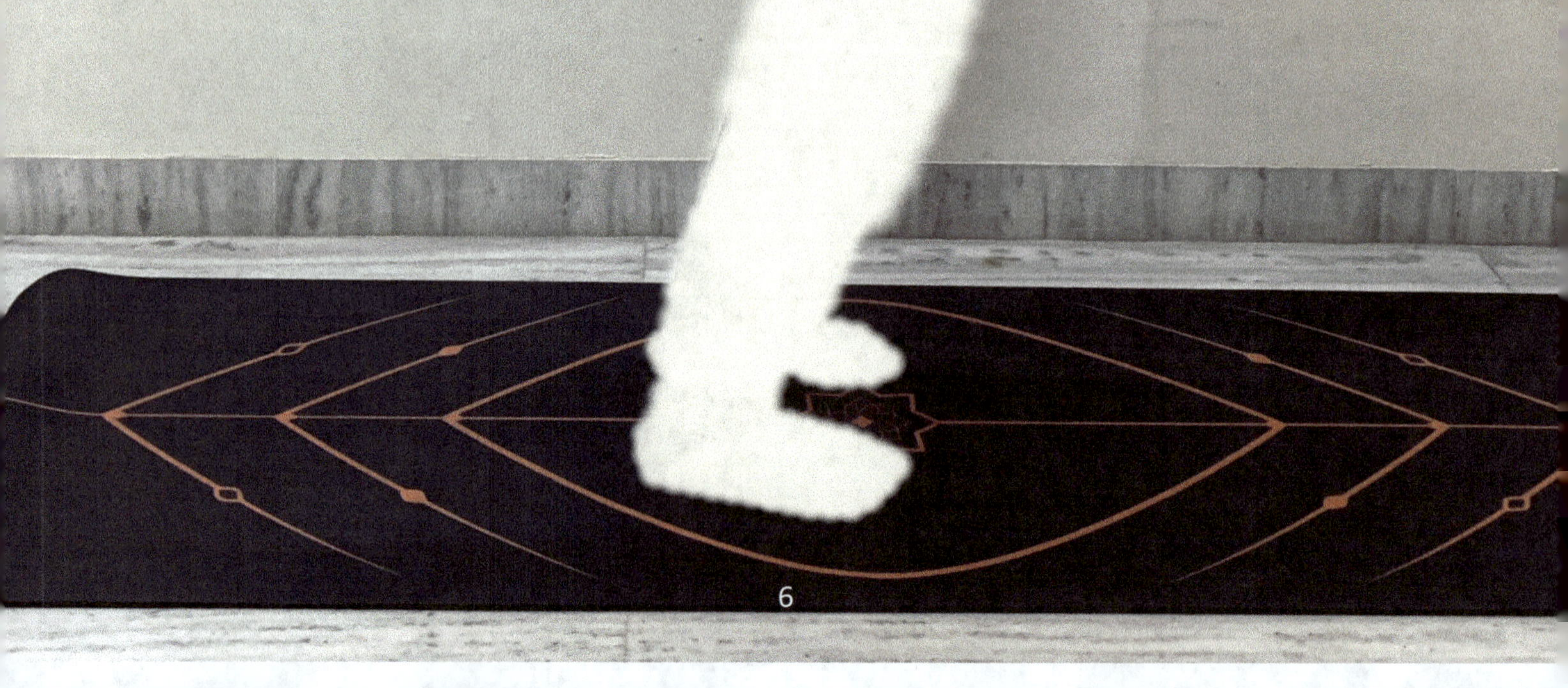

What is Yoga

Yoga is a higher state of Being. It is a state of the consciousness that reflects Purity, Cheerfulness, Compassion. Yoga is that moment in life when one is at ease, absorbed in divine union.

The entire process that comprises of

- Shouldering Responsibility Well,
- Taking Timely Action,
- Making Wise Decisions,
- Handling Difficult Situations, and Displaying
- Grit, Humility, Patience and Perseverance

this entire process is another name for the Practice of Yoga.
The methods and techniques given in this book are a means to achieve the DIVINE UNION = SWEET BLISS = YOGA.

This is made possible by treading the Path of Yoga.

Etymology

In Sanskrit, there is a Root (Dhatu or primary sound) named युज् । It belongs to the 7th Conjugational Group. Its Dhatu Serial Number is 1444.

युजिर् योगे । Entry as listed in the Dhatupatha of Panini.
Using various Affixes, we are able to form the following words.
युज् + घञ् -> योग । Joining, Union, Dissolving, Becoming One.
युज् + घञ् -> योग + सुँ -> योगः । Actual spelling of Yoga used when writing a Sanskrit sentence.
युज् + घिनुण् -> योगिन् । A Yogi. One who is absorbed in the Divine.
युज् + क्त -> युक्त । Appropriate. Befitting.

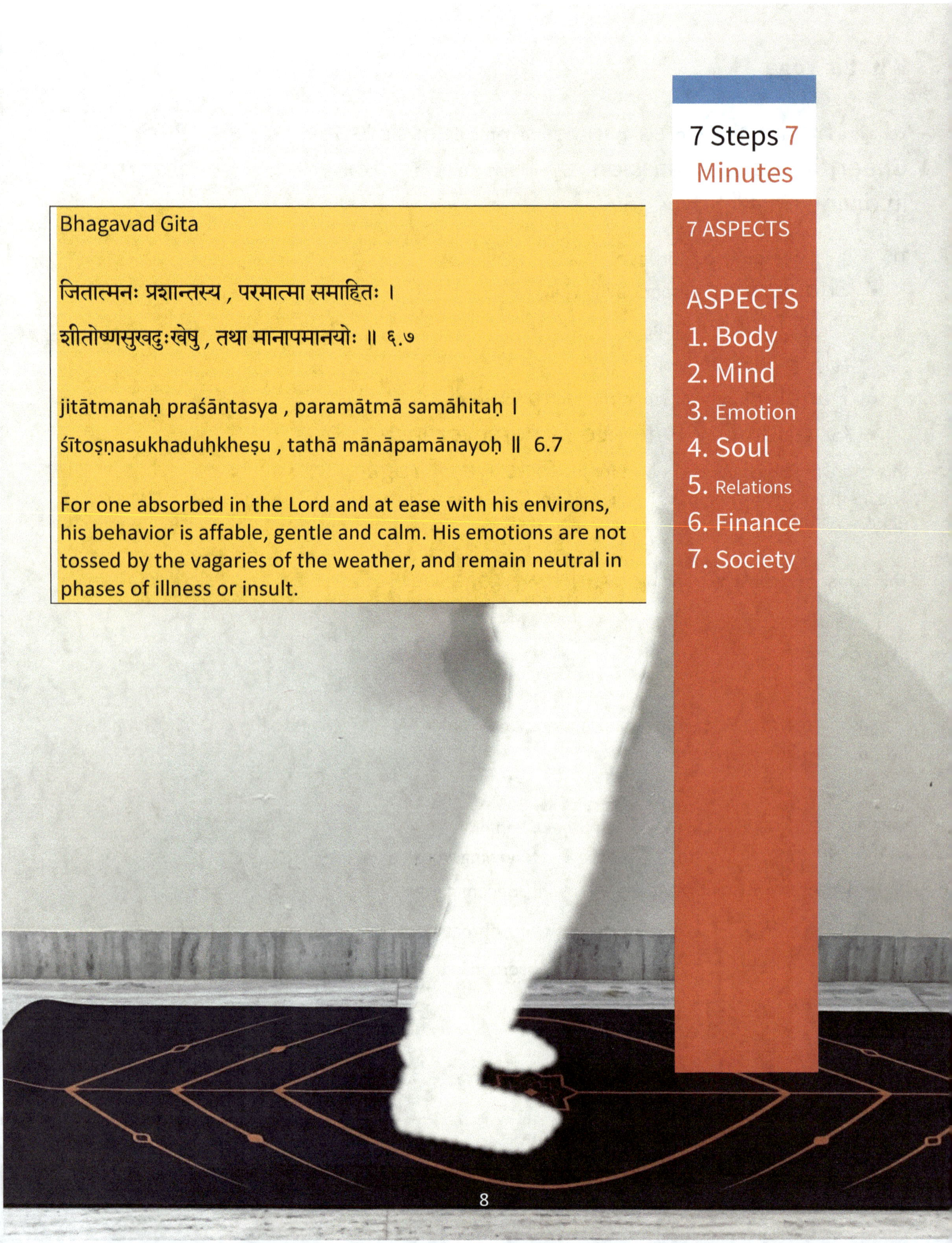

Bhagavad Gita

जितात्मनः प्रशान्तस्य , परमात्मा समाहितः ।

शीतोष्णसुखदुःखेषु , तथा मानापमानयोः ॥ ६.७

jitātmanaḥ praśāntasya , paramātmā samāhitaḥ I

śītoṣṇasukhaduḥkheṣu , tathā mānāpamānayoḥ II 6.7

For one absorbed in the Lord and at ease with his environs, his behavior is affable, gentle and calm. His emotions are not tossed by the vagaries of the weather, and remain neutral in phases of illness or insult.

ASPECTS

1. Body
2. Mind
3. Emotion
4. Soul
5. Relations
6. Finance
7. Society

Props deepen the Yoga Experience

A Yoga drill can be made interesting, safe, inventive and beneficial according to our comfort level and body state, by means of simple equipment that are present in every home.

Yoga Mat & Water Bottle

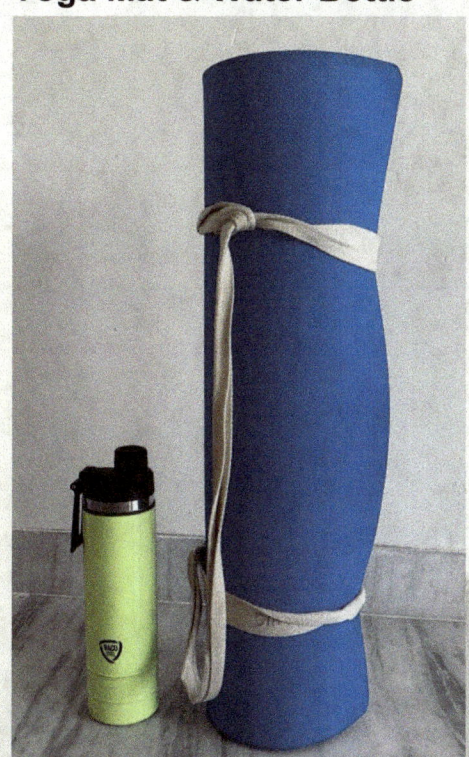

a good Yoga Mat enhances our practice and is a must since
it does not slip,
prevents knee and ankle strain,
prevents cold floor,
absorbs perspiration,
gives haptic feedback.

Pillow, Folded Bath Towel

We can tuck it under our ankles or use it for sitting on during Vajrasana and use it under our neck for specific postures.

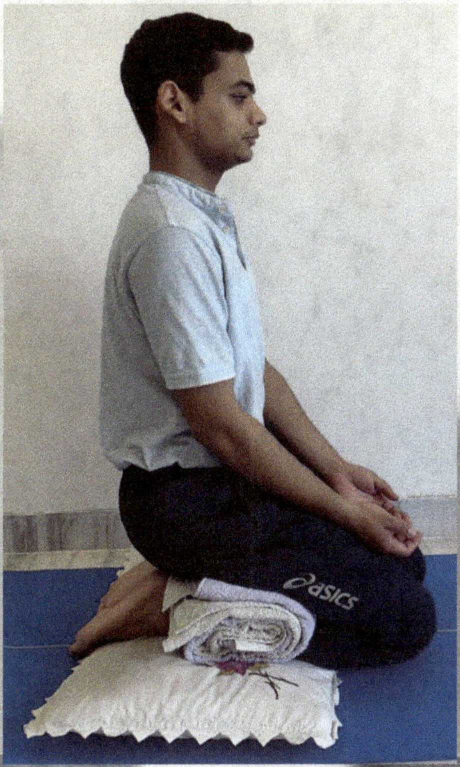

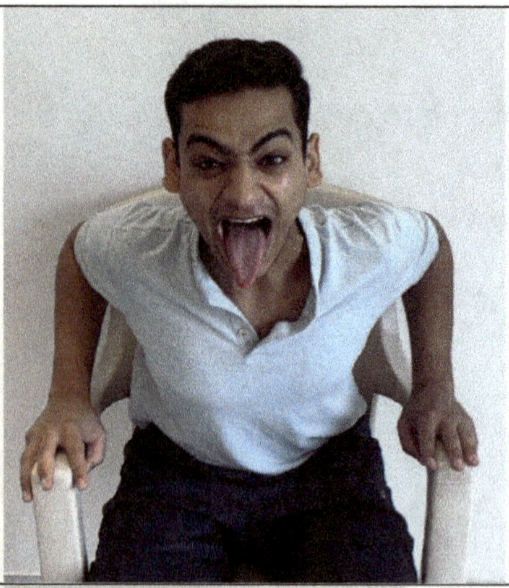

Chair with Armrest

A chair with armrest comes in handy when we are doing Agnisar Kriya or Simhasana, as it helps to make the body tension appropriate.

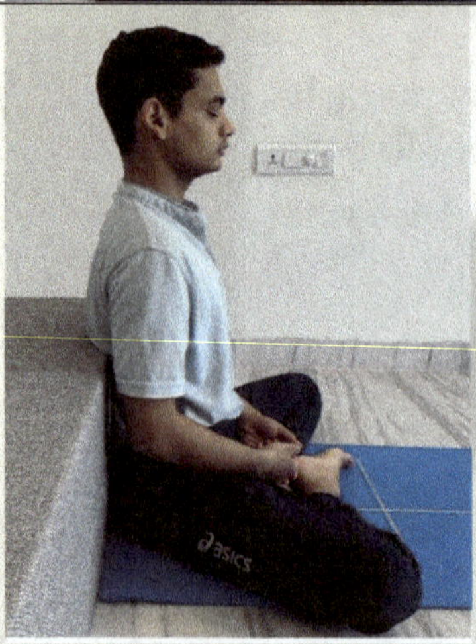

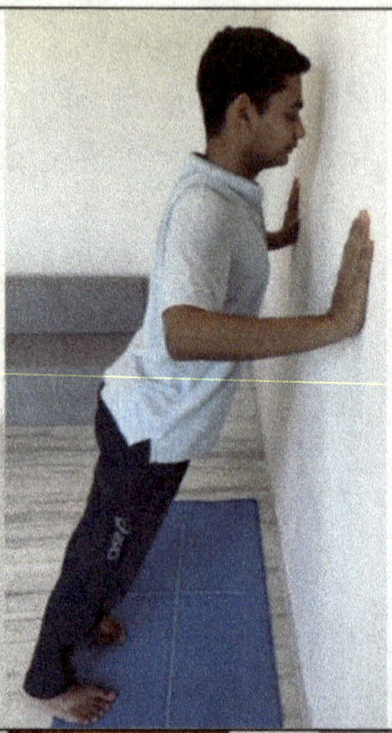

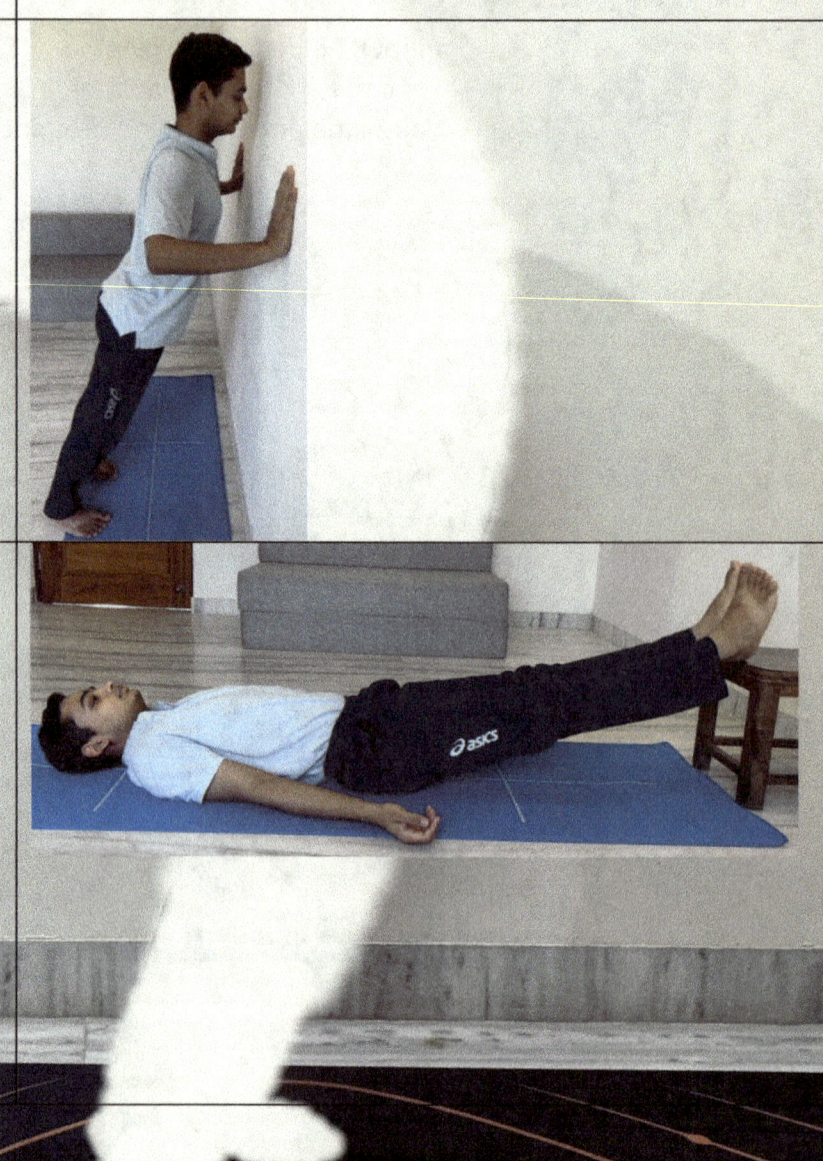

Chair without Armrest

A chair can help in proper backrest during Meditation or some sitting postures. Especially during Bhastrika, a chair without armrest can be used.

Wall

A dead wall can be safely used to aid various postures, also as a backrest.

Bench

At times a bench or stool comes in handy for push-ups and similar postures.

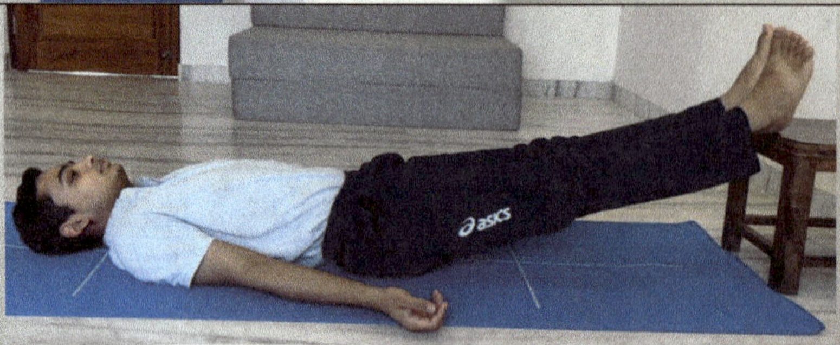

Yogacharya's Grace

Supreme Guide, Superlative Teaching

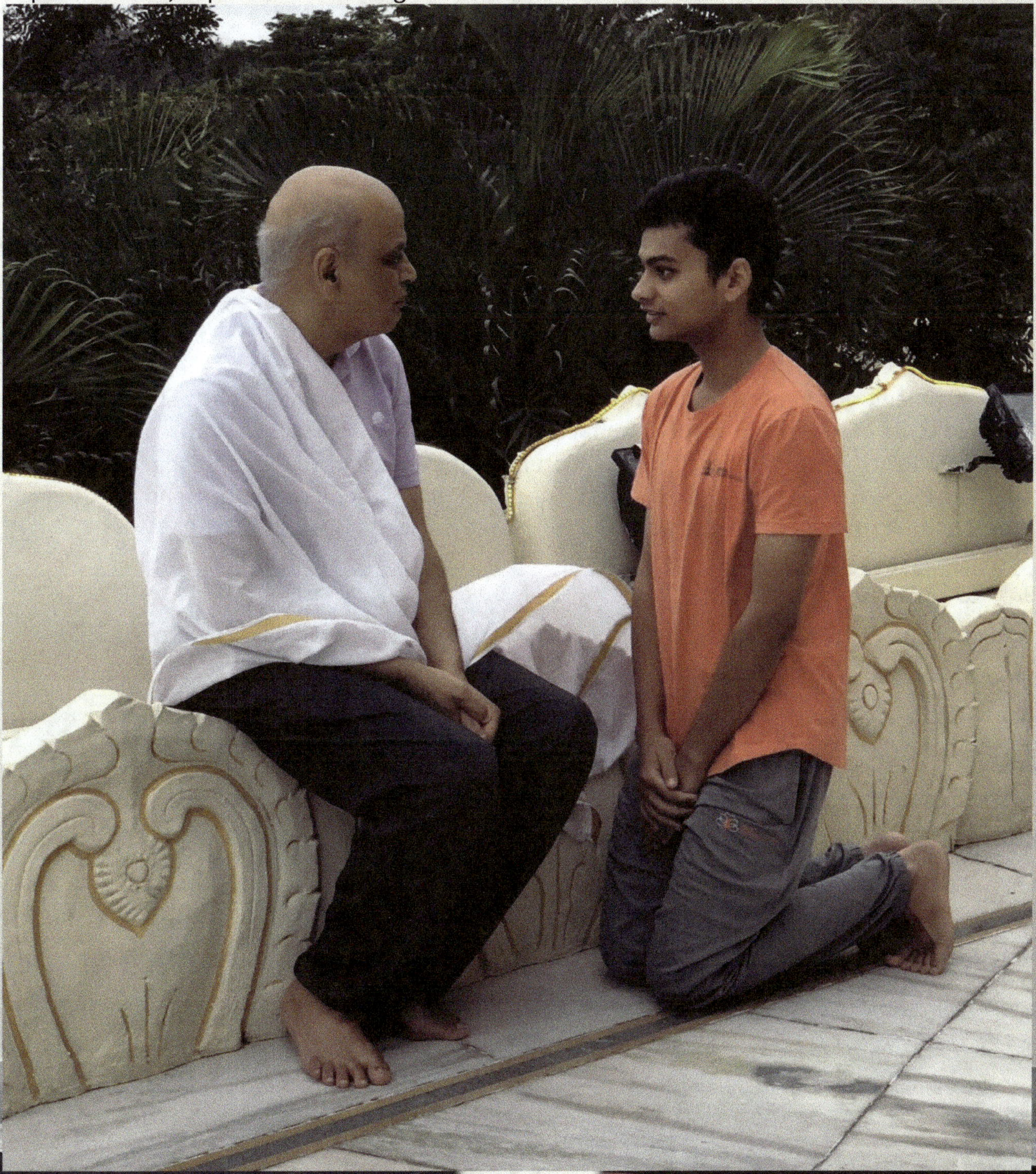

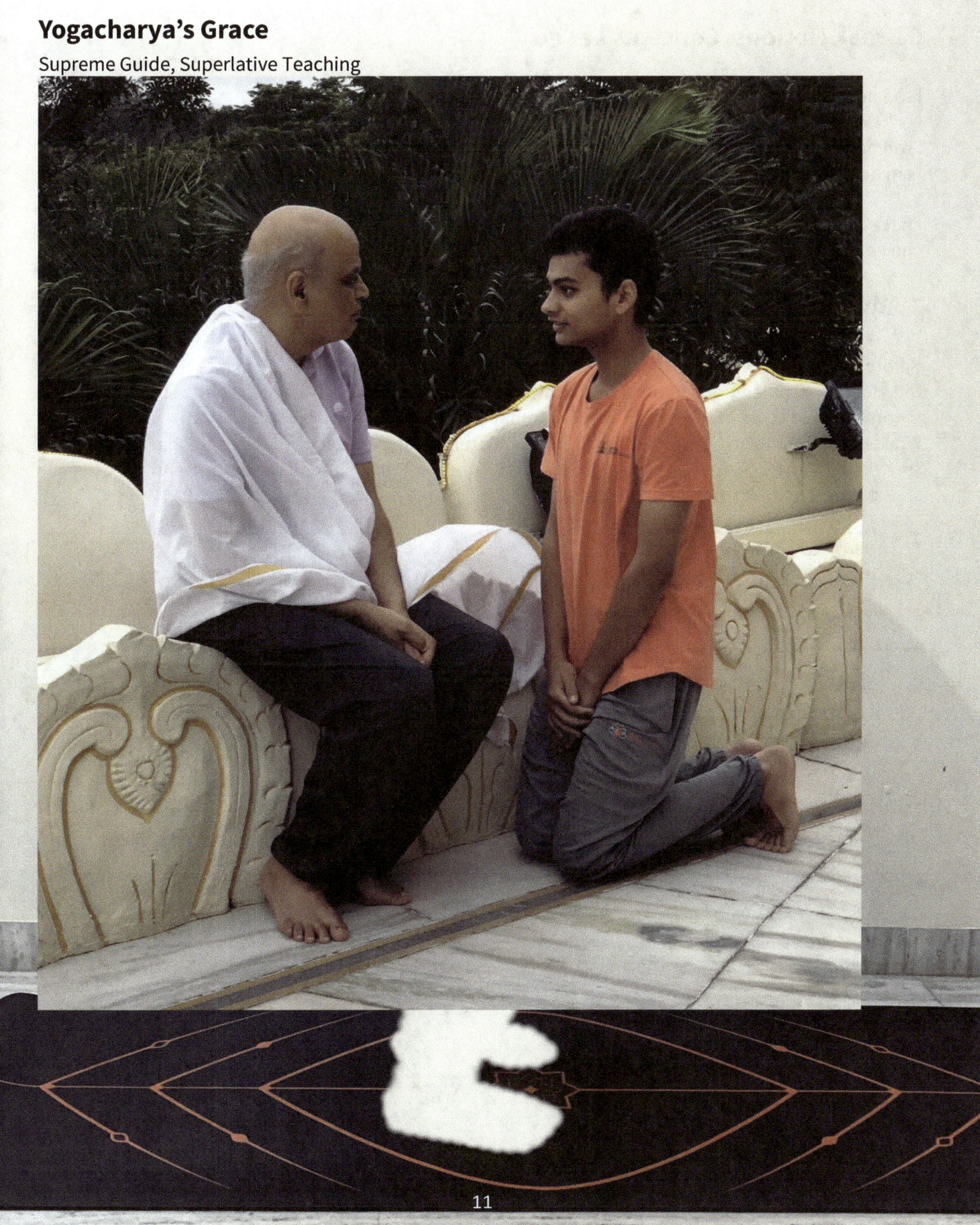

0 Break Notions, Concepts Let go

I will do Yoga only in the morning.
I will do Yoga only after finishing my work.
I will do Yoga on the weekends.
I am doing Advanced Courses once a year, that is enough.

I have my Master's grace, what else? My dear, life itself is grace. Each moment well-lived is a conscious choice, made with determination, sincerity, self-will.

1 Advanced Postures

Before we start serious asana practice, it is a good idea to do simple warm ups to awaken and activate the muscles, ligaments and joints. This can prevent injury and make the asana results better. **It is recommended to do asanas on an empty stomach, preferably 3 hours after a meal.**
When one begins to enjoy asana practice, it is but natural that the fitter or younger amongst us would seek something more. Here are some of our favorite asanas. It makes good sense to attend a yoga studio in person to learn and hone these postures.

PATANJALI YOGA SUTRA

स्थिर–सुखम् आसनम् ॥ sthirasukhamāsanam ॥ 2.46 ॥

2.46 Asana is that which is Stable and Comfortable

ततः क्षीयते प्रकाश–आवरणम् ॥ २.५२ ॥ tataḥ kṣīyate prakāśāvaraṇam ॥ 2.52 ॥

2.52 Then the veil on the Light becomes worn-out

By the practice of Pranayama the veil that covers the Soul gets tattered. Breath Control as learnt from a Master and practiced willingly removes the mask that obscures the Divinity within us.

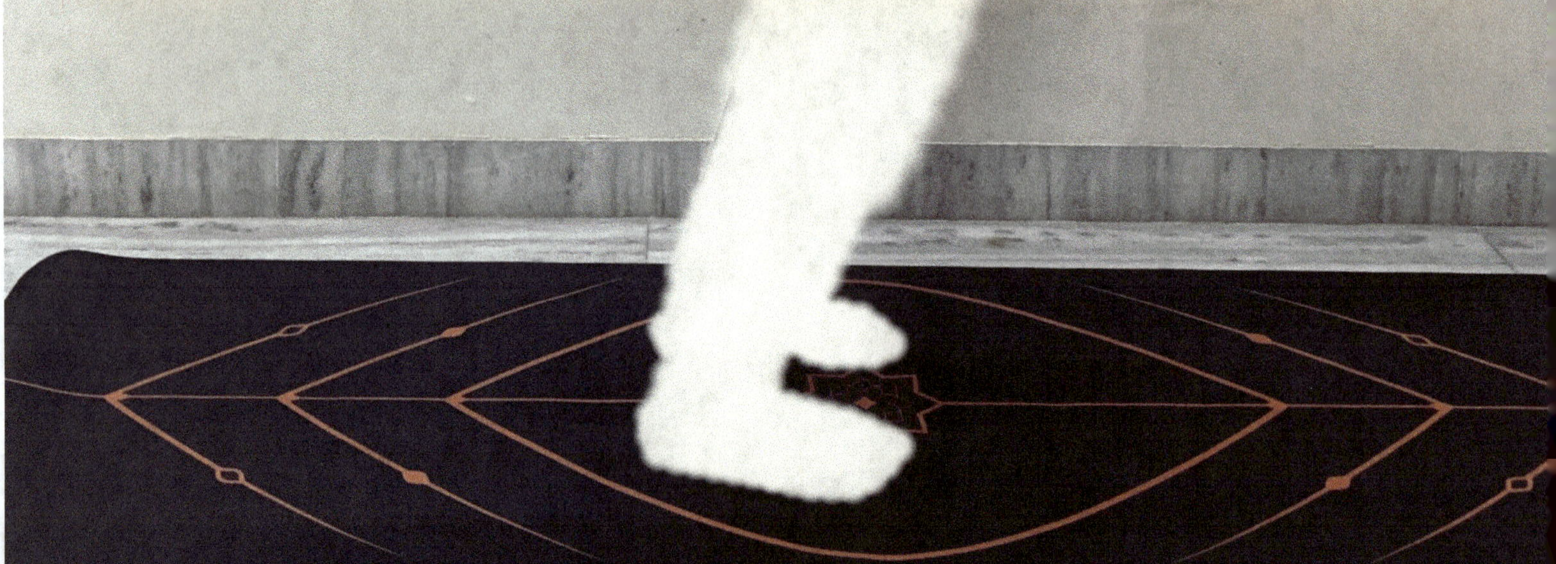

Lotus Pose - Padmāsana

MIND WHAT'S HAPPENING
Rather light in the head, not so many thoughts.

BODY WHERE IS THE EFFECT
Central Nervous System.

ATTENTION
On the third eye, ajna chakra.

BREATH
Smooth and Natural breathing.

SEQUENCE

- Sit down on the floor. Lift the right foot with both hands and place it on the left thigh. Adjust for comfort.
- Now lift the left foot and place it on the right thigh.
- Rock a bit and adjust for comfort.
- Keep both hands on the knees on in the lap.
- Bring the awareness in between the eyebrows
- Breathe naturally.

On alternate days, we can reverse the leg position, i.e. left leg below and right leg on top.

COUNTER POSE = Butterfly and cradling the baby.

ASPECTS
1. Body
2. Mind
3. Emotion
4. Soul
5. Relations
6. Finance
7. Society

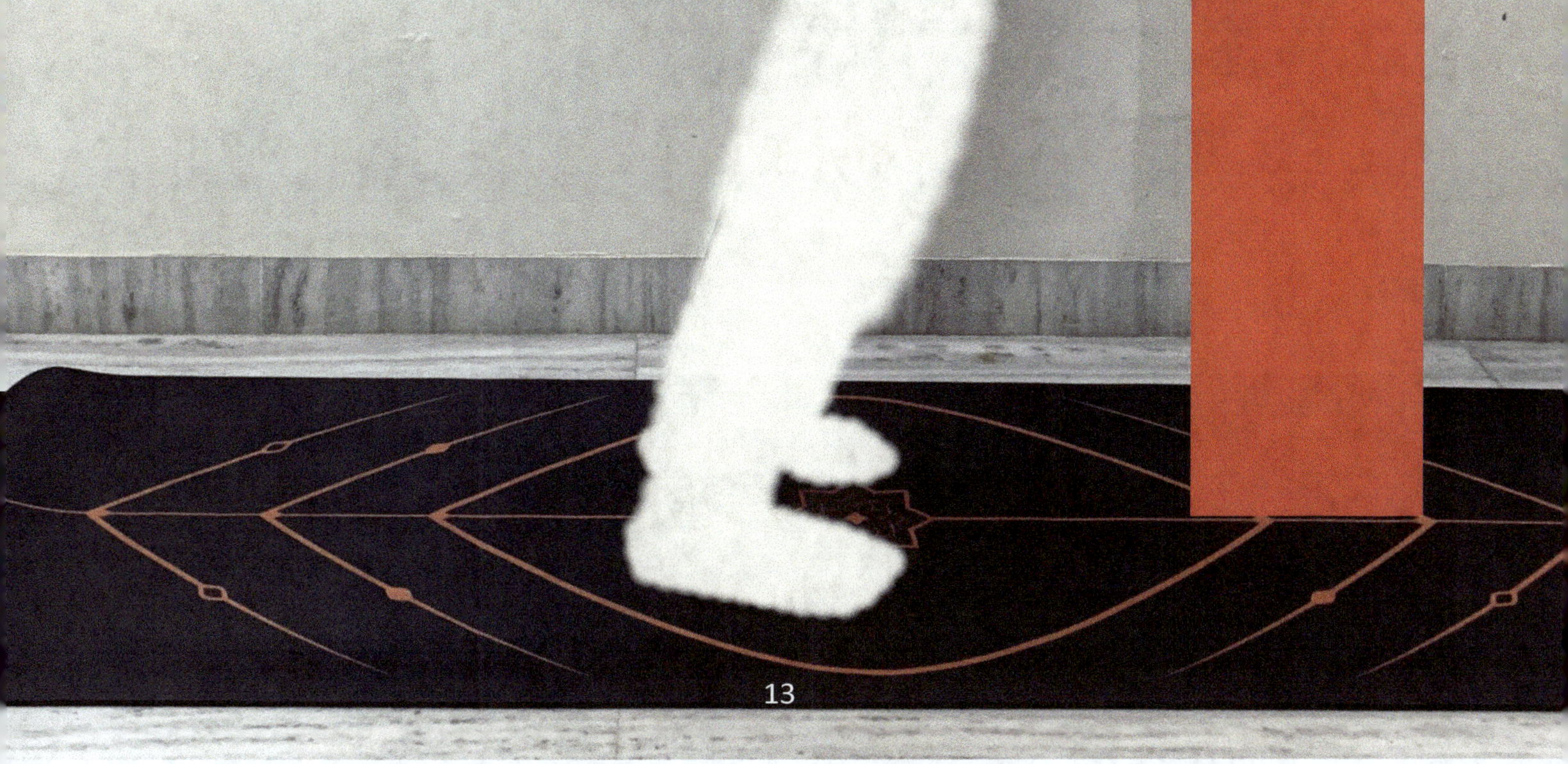

LOTUS

PADMASANA

LIGHT GRACE FUL

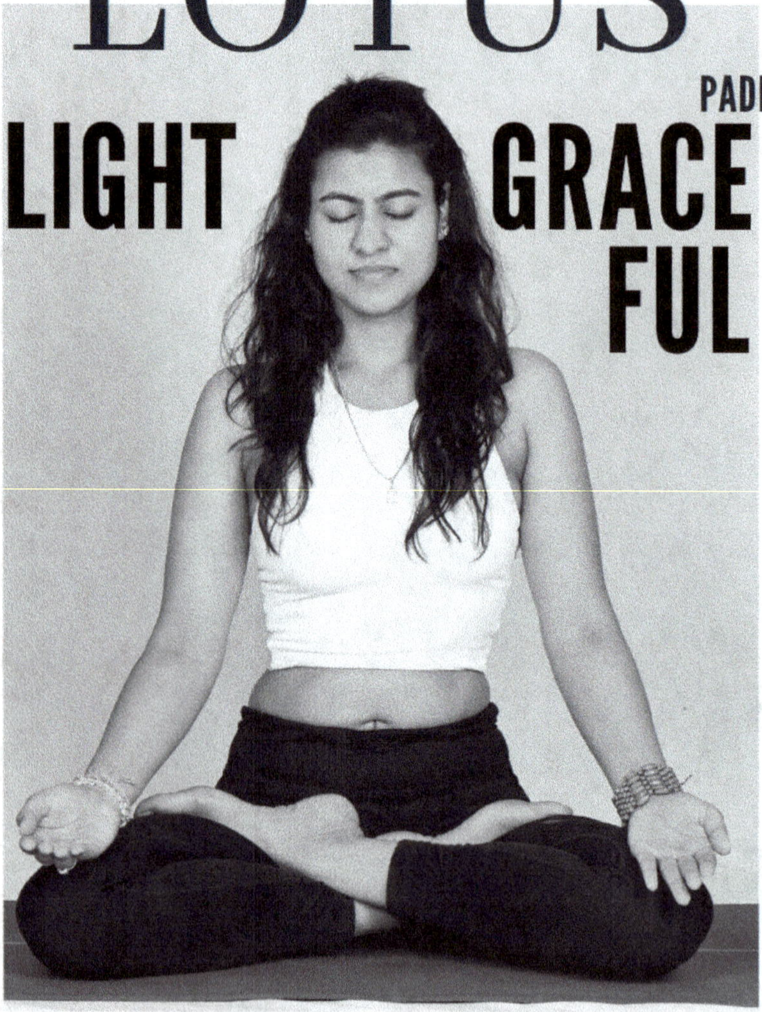

INWARD EYE OUTWARD SUCCESS

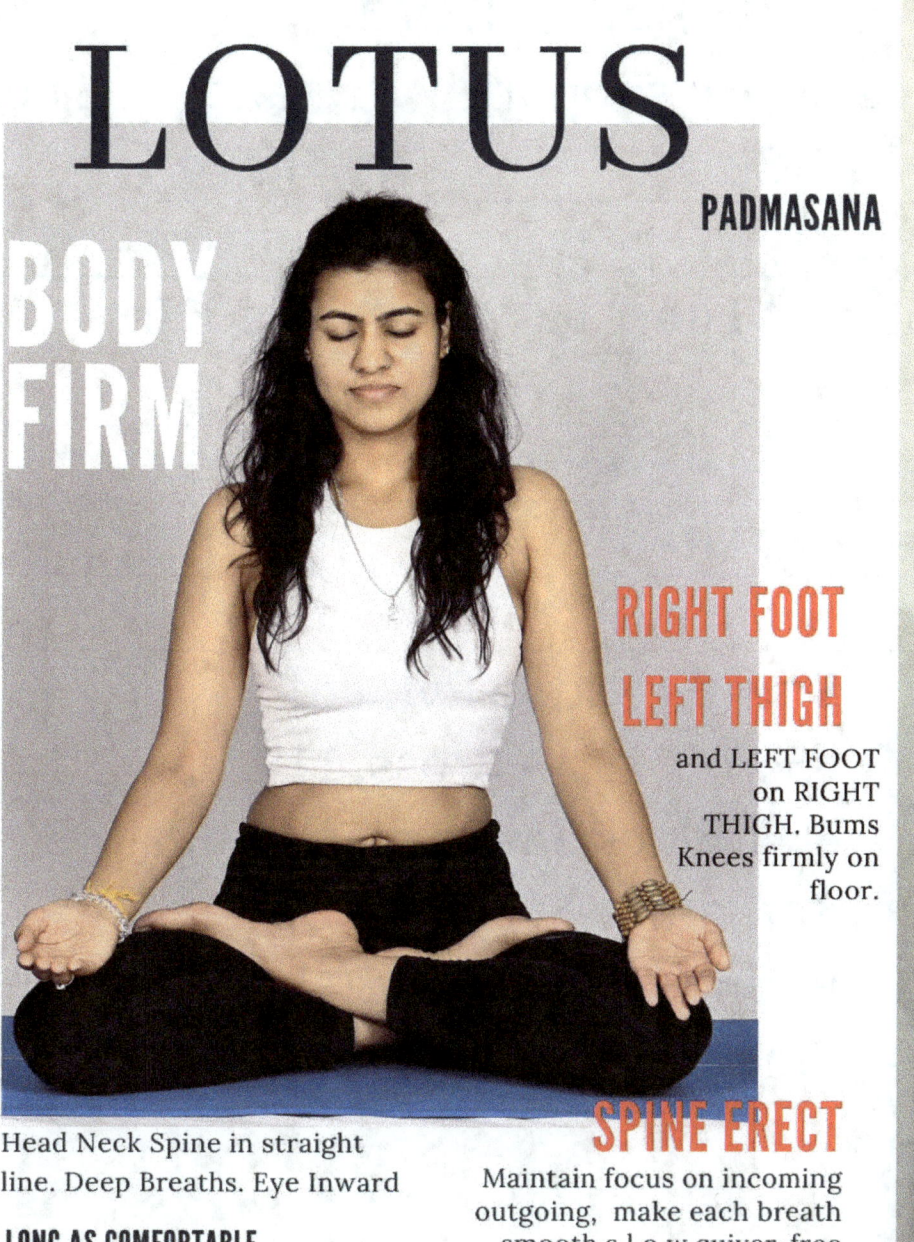

LOTUS

PADMASANA

BODY FIRM

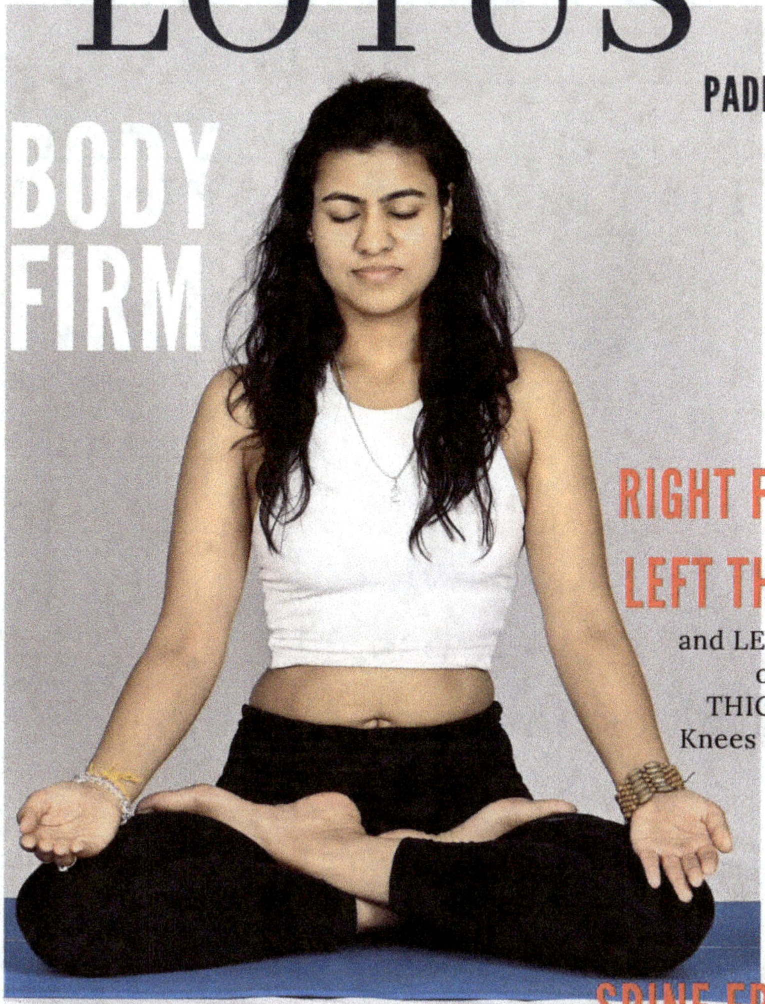

RIGHT FOOT LEFT THIGH

and LEFT FOOT on RIGHT THIGH. Bums Knees firmly on floor.

Head Neck Spine in straight line. Deep Breaths. Eye Inward

POSE AS LONG AS COMFORTABLE

SPINE ERECT

Maintain focus on incoming outgoing, make each breath smooth s l o w quiver-free

https://www.srisritattva.com/

Sri Sri Tattva A Health Juice Duo to support cardio and joint health		
Product	Size	Price
Cardio Tonic	Common	India
Arjuna Garcinia Juice	1 Liter	Rs 320
Joint Mobility	Common	India
Artho Fix Juice	1 Liter	Rs 400
India wide Shipping		

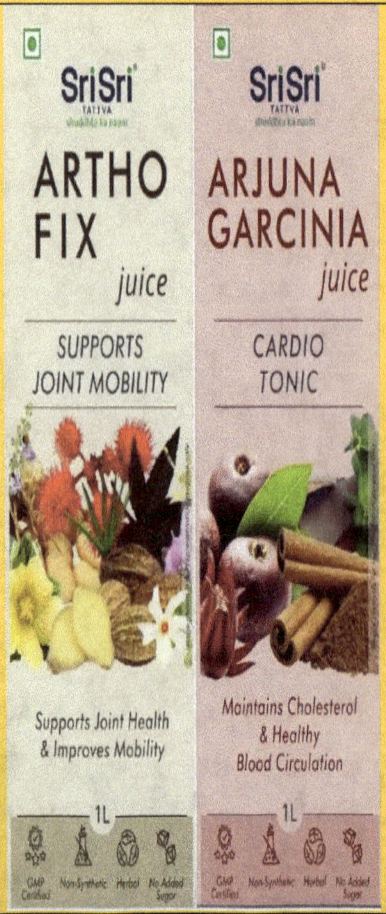

Sriveda Sattva Pvt. Ltd.
#54/56, 39th A Cross, 11th Main,
4th T Block Jayanagar, Bengaluru
Karnataka 560041 INDIA
Phone 1800 120 8030
Email onlinesupport@srisritattva.com

Back Stretch - Paschimottanāsana

MIND WHAT'S HAPPENING
Rather tense initially, but relaxes later on.

BODY WHERE IS THE EFFECT
Spine, Thighs, Knees, Calves, Feet.

ATTENTION

- On the keeping the back muscles relaxed.
- In the genital area – the Swadhisthana Chakra.

BREATH

- Inhale while you raise your arms up.
- Exhale while bending forward.
- Keep breathing in the posture.
- Inhale while straightening up.

SEQUENCE

- Sit on the floor with your legs stretched out in the front.
- Pull out the fleshy parts of your hips with the help of your hands and sit on your sitting bones.
- Raise both your arms and stretch your torso up.
- Bend forward with your chest pushing out.
- Take your arms towards the front wall, and the chest towards the legs. Keep your head straight.
- Pull your abdomen in, and drop your arms on the legs wherever you can reach.
- Grab the legs, bend the elbows and pull yourself further into the stretch.
- Drop your chest and head. Close your eyes.
- To come out of the posture, slide your arms back on the legs and gently straighten your spine.

- COUNTER POSE = Bhujangasana Cobra

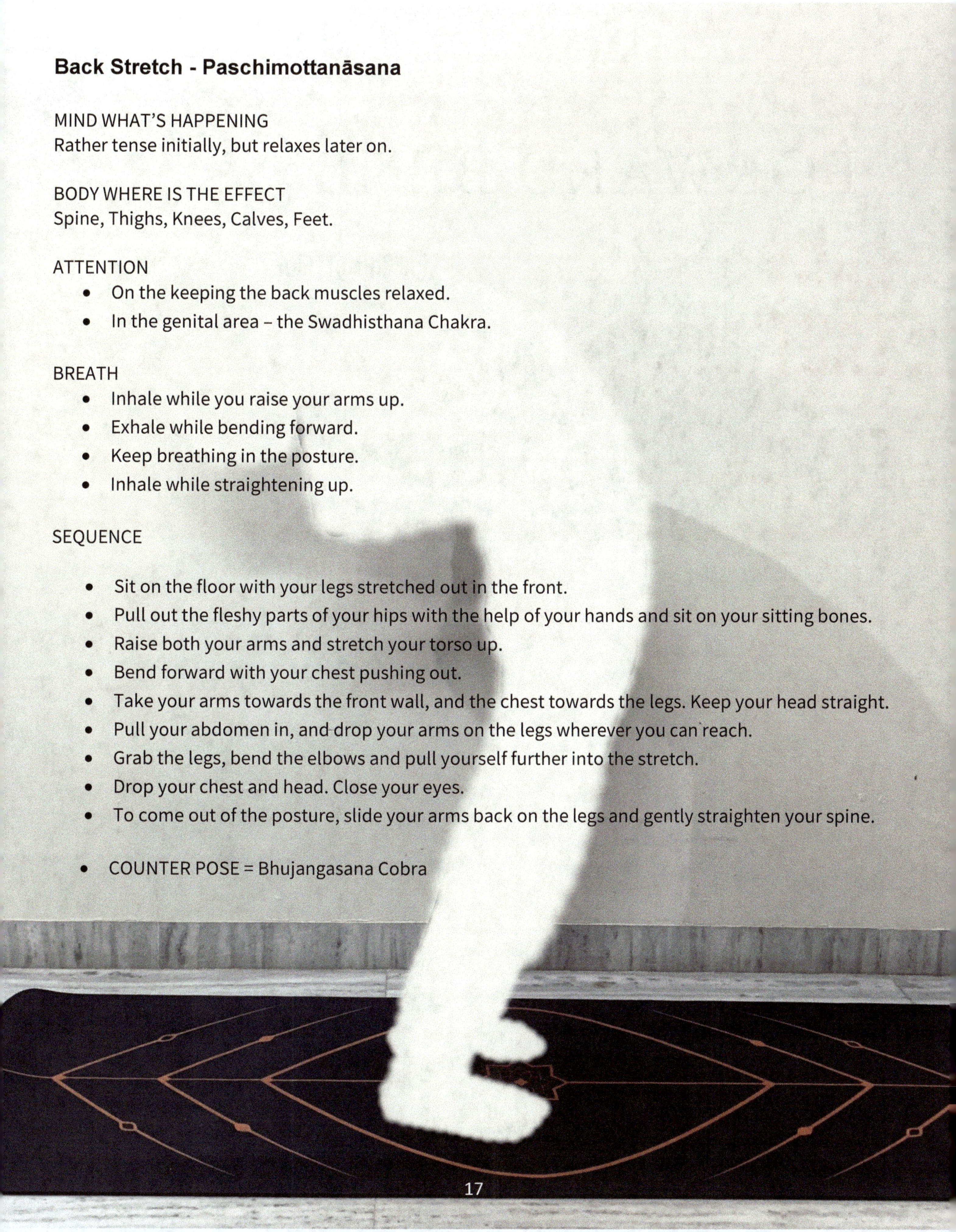

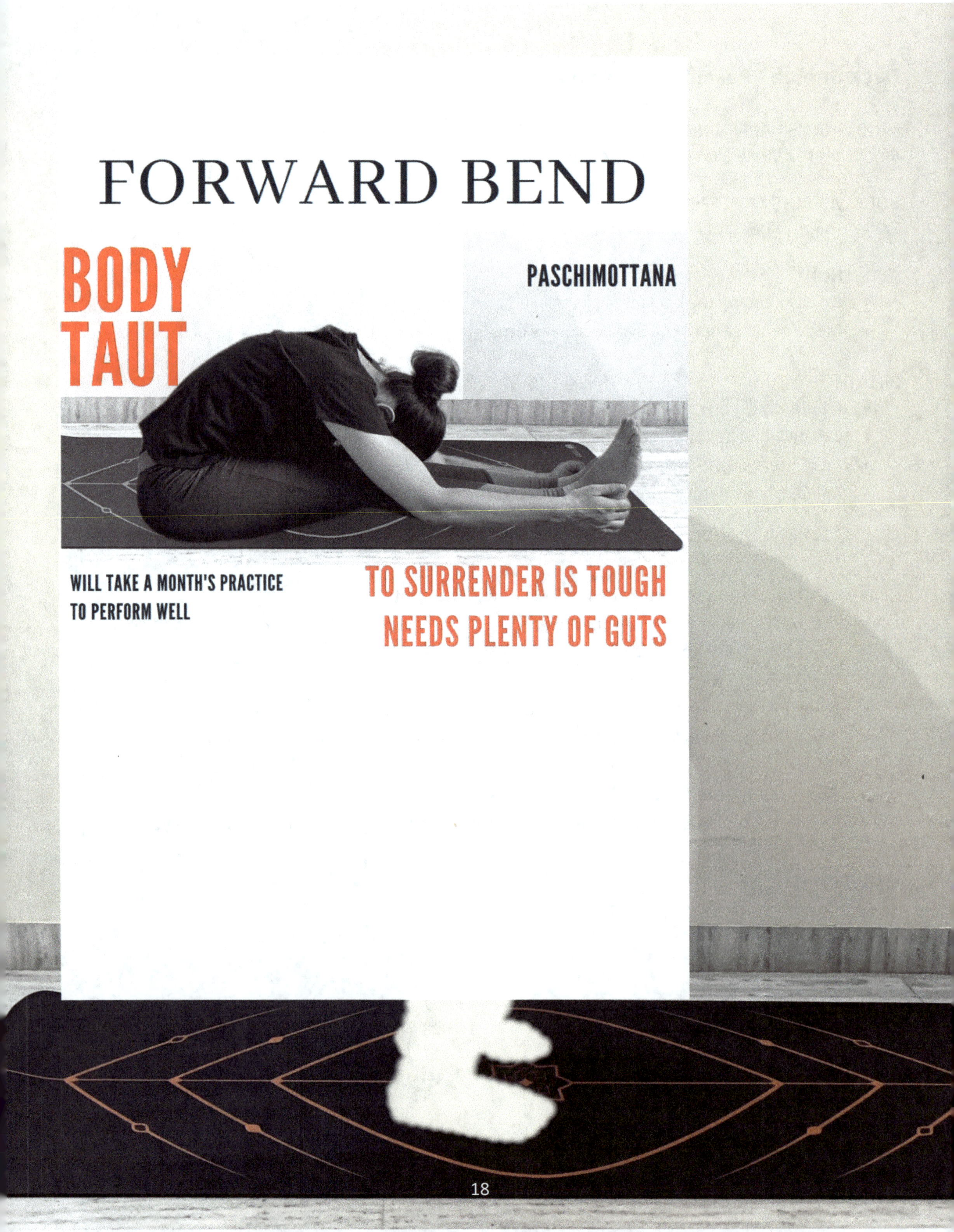

FORWARD BEND

BODY TAUT

PASCHIMOTTANA

WILL TAKE A MONTH'S PRACTICE TO PERFORM WELL

TO SURRENDER IS TOUGH
NEEDS PLENTY OF GUTS

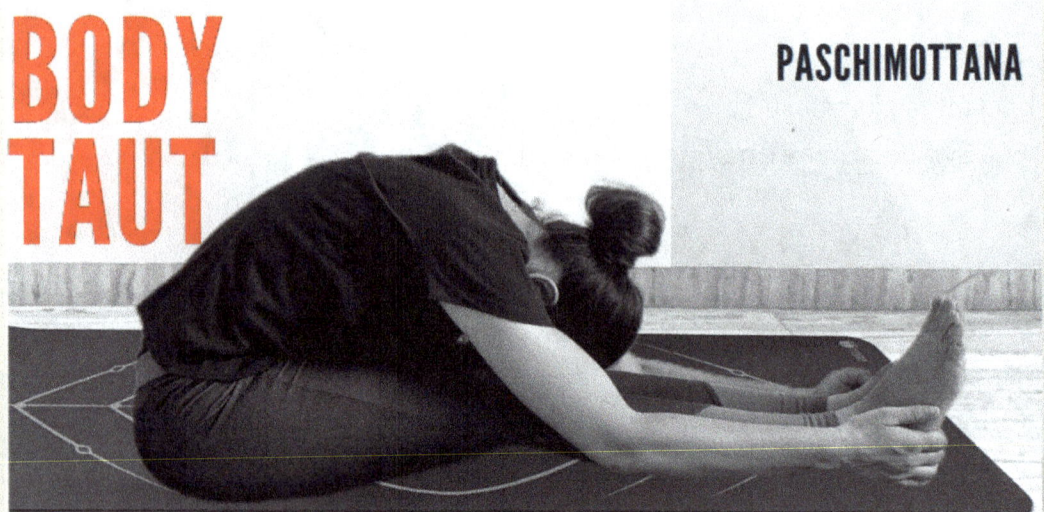

FORWARD BEND

7 Steps 7 Minutes

7 ASPECTS

STEPS
1. Asana
2. Breath
3. Walk
4. Meditation
5. Bath
6. Havan
7. Sports

PASCHIMOTTANA

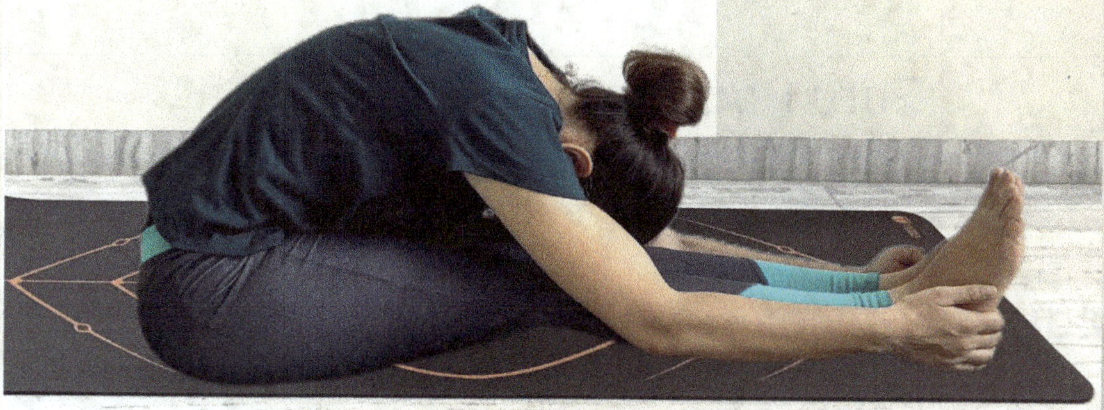

SLOW BEND, HEAD TO KNEES

Lift slowly forward from a lying down position

CATCH YOUR FEET

Needs plenty of focus, make each breath smooth s l o w quiver-free

POSE AS LONG AS COMFORTABLE

https://www.artofliving.org/

The Art of Living Programs, Events, Endeavors for All		
Happiness Course	Advanced Meditation Course	Sri Sri Yoga
Intuition Process	Sahaj Samadhi	Art Excel Course
Shivratri Celebrations	Guru Poornima Celebrations	Navratri Celebrations
Organic Farming	Desi Cow Goshala	Cold Pressed Oils
Ayurveda Nadi Pariksha	Pancakarma Oil Massage	Marma Therapy
Satsang	Guru Puja	Teacher Training
Schools	Colleges	University
Worldwide Presence in 180 Countries		

The Art of Living International Center
21st Km Kanakapura Road, Udayapura,
Bengaluru, Karnataka 560082 INDIA
Landline +91 80 67262626
Email info@vvmvp.org
https://twitter.com/bangaloreashram

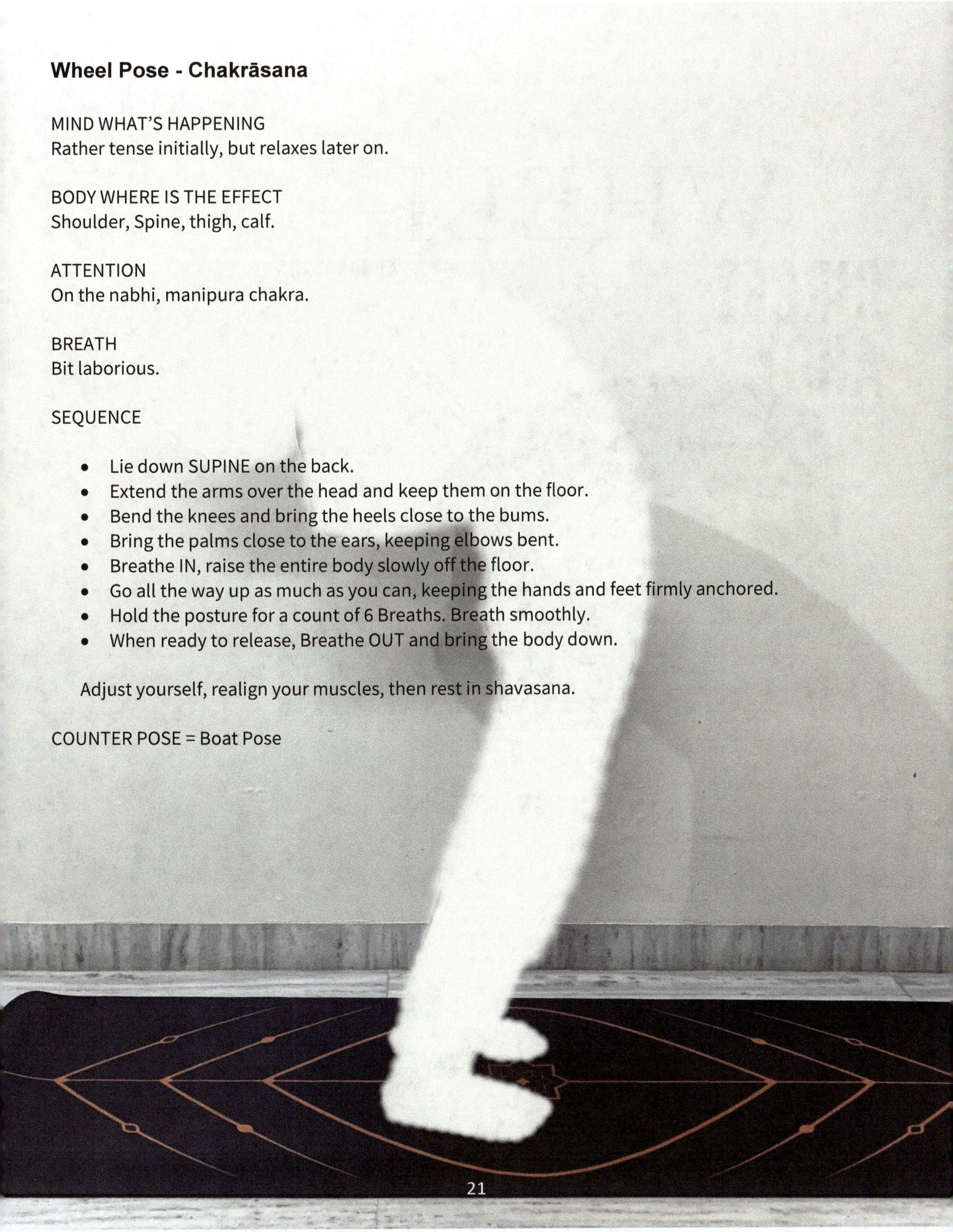

Wheel Pose - Chakrāsana

MIND WHAT'S HAPPENING
Rather tense initially, but relaxes later on.

BODY WHERE IS THE EFFECT
Shoulder, Spine, thigh, calf.

ATTENTION
On the nabhi, manipura chakra.

BREATH
Bit laborious.

SEQUENCE

- Lie down SUPINE on the back.
- Extend the arms over the head and keep them on the floor.
- Bend the knees and bring the heels close to the bums.
- Bring the palms close to the ears, keeping elbows bent.
- Breathe IN, raise the entire body slowly off the floor.
- Go all the way up as much as you can, keeping the hands and feet firmly anchored.
- Hold the posture for a count of 6 Breaths. Breath smoothly.
- When ready to release, Breathe OUT and bring the body down.

Adjust yourself, realign your muscles, then rest in shavasana.

COUNTER POSE = Boat Pose

WHEEL

CHAKRASANA

CIRCLE AHOY

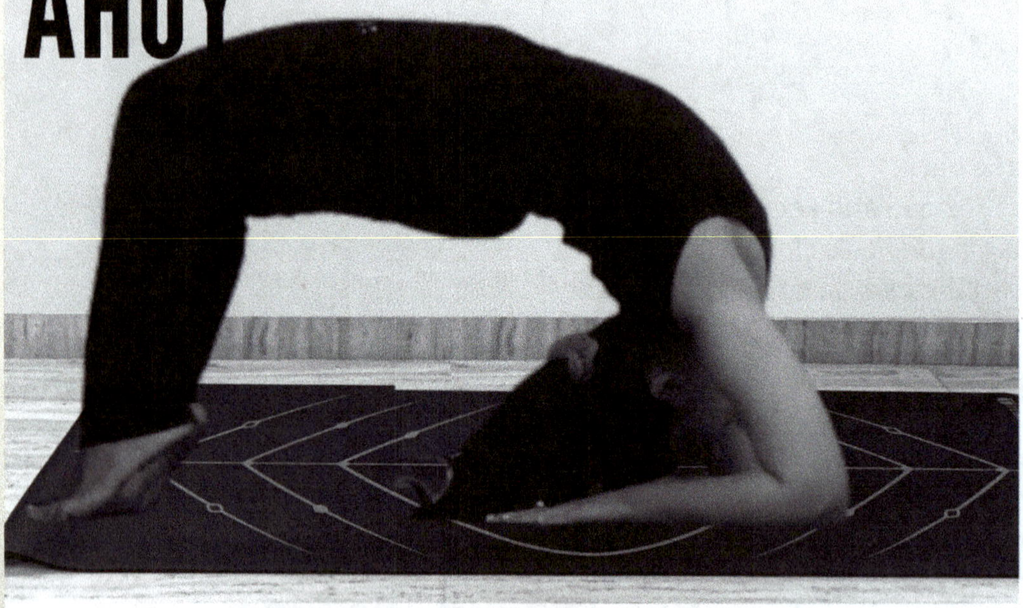

WHEN THE MIND BECOMES FLEXIBLE

I CAN CARTWHEEL

ADVANCED POSE - UNDER SUPERVISION

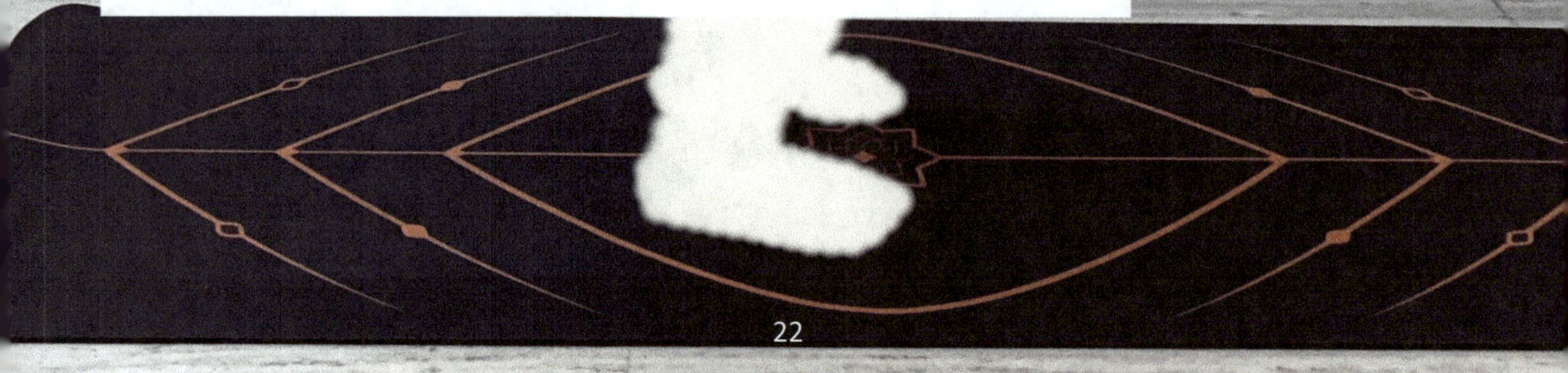

WHEEL

CHAKRASANA

BODY FIRM

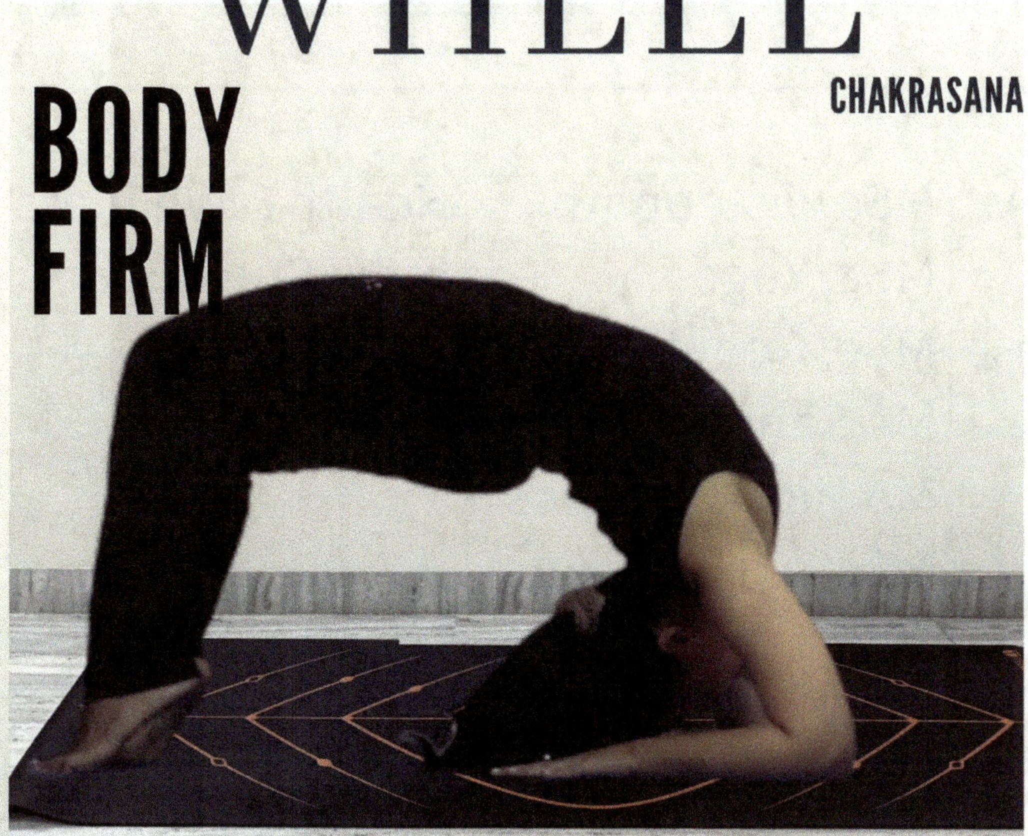

A nice lift of the Torso.
Feet shoulder-width apart.
Neck steady

PALMS INWARD

Shoulders Firm, Chest Out

NECK FIRM

Maintain Focus on lower back,
Make each breath smooth s l o w
quiver-free

POSE FOR 6 BREATHS

Tree - Vrikshāsana

MIND WHAT'S HAPPENING
Rather light in the head, not so many thoughts.

BODY WHERE IS THE EFFECT
Neck, Spine, abdomen, pelvis, and hips.

ATTENTION

- On the leg which is on the floor, the chest, head and arms.
- Focus on the breath to keep it tremor free.
- On the eyebrow center – the Ajna Chakra.

BREATH

- Inhale while raising the arms up.
- Inhale and then place the right foot on the left thigh.
- Keep breathing in the posture.
- Inhale while placing the right foot back on the floor.
- Exhale while lowering the arms down.

SEQUENCE

- Stand straight with feet hip-width apart.
- Balance your body equally on both feet.
- Tuck in the tailbone; pull the abdomen in; push the chest out; take the chin slightly towards the chest.
- Raise both arms up over the head and join the hands in a Namaste.
- Fix your gaze in front; raise the right knee and place the right foot on the left thigh close to the groin above the knee.
- Close your eyes if balance can be maintained.
- To come out of the posture, put down the right foot back on the floor and then bring the arms down.

COUNTER POSE = Other Leg

7Minutes In just 7 minutes a day, do 1 Step of your favorite practice.

And see the result in 7 days

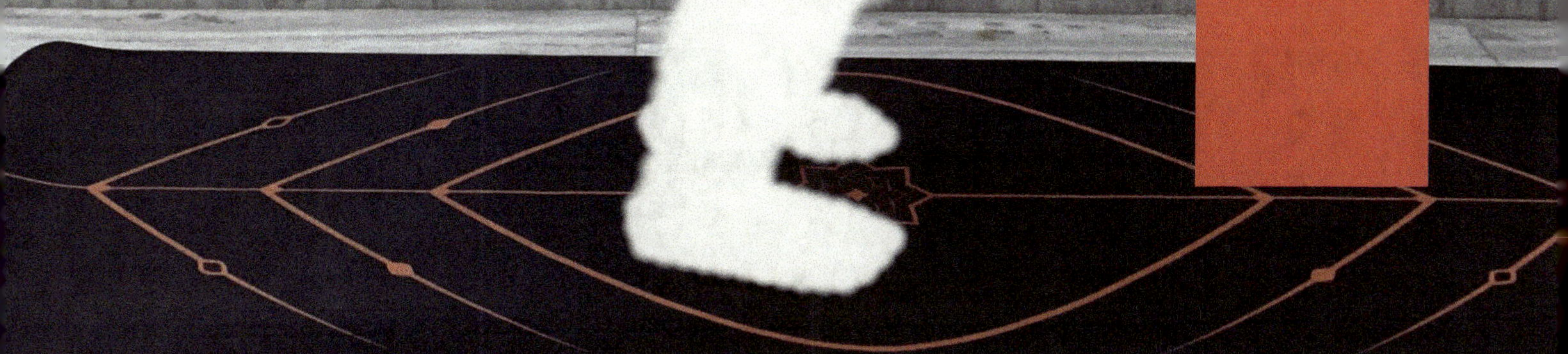

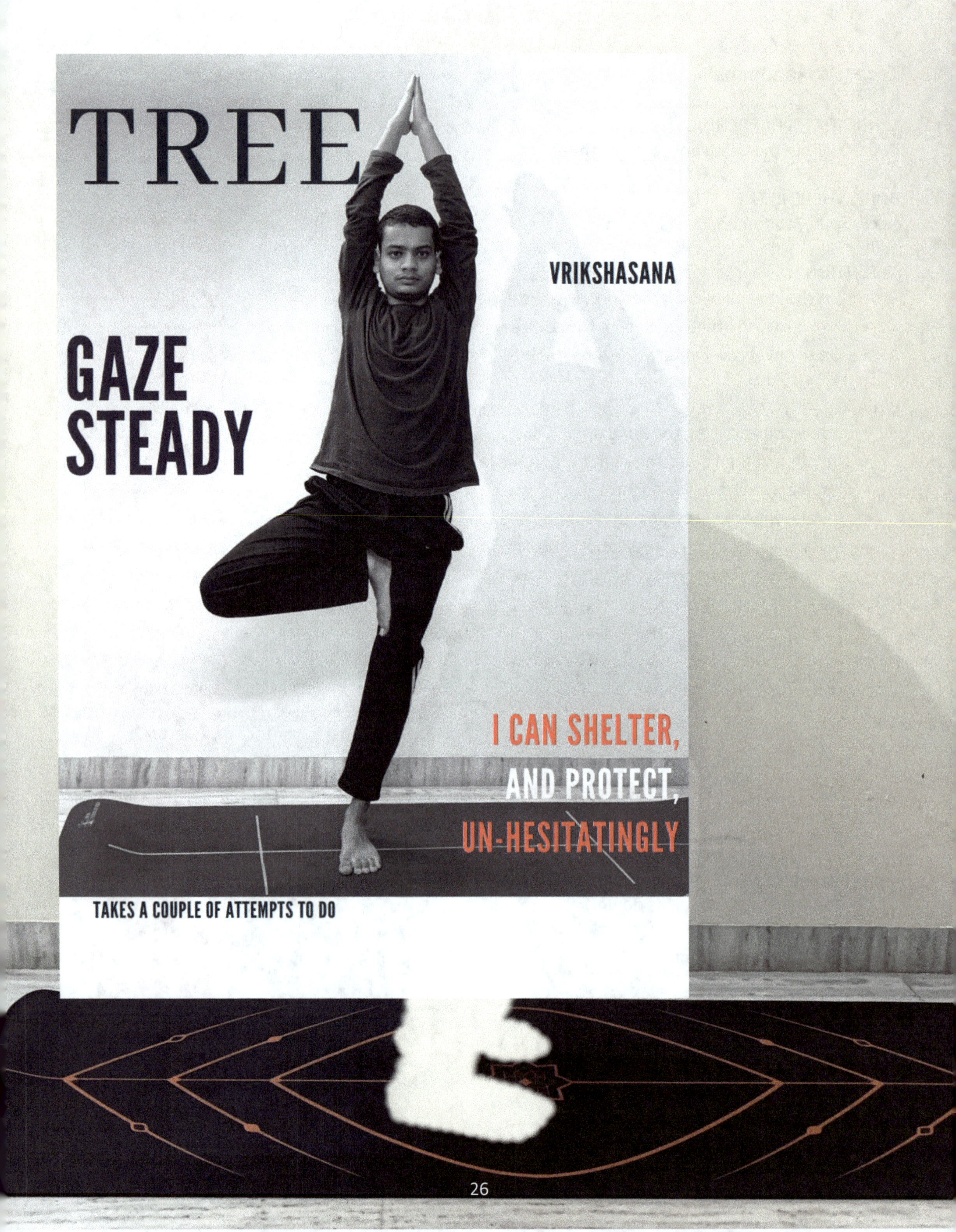

TREE

VRIKSHASANA

GAZE STEADY

I CAN SHELTER,
AND PROTECT,
UN-HESITATINGLY

TAKES A COUPLE OF ATTEMPTS TO DO

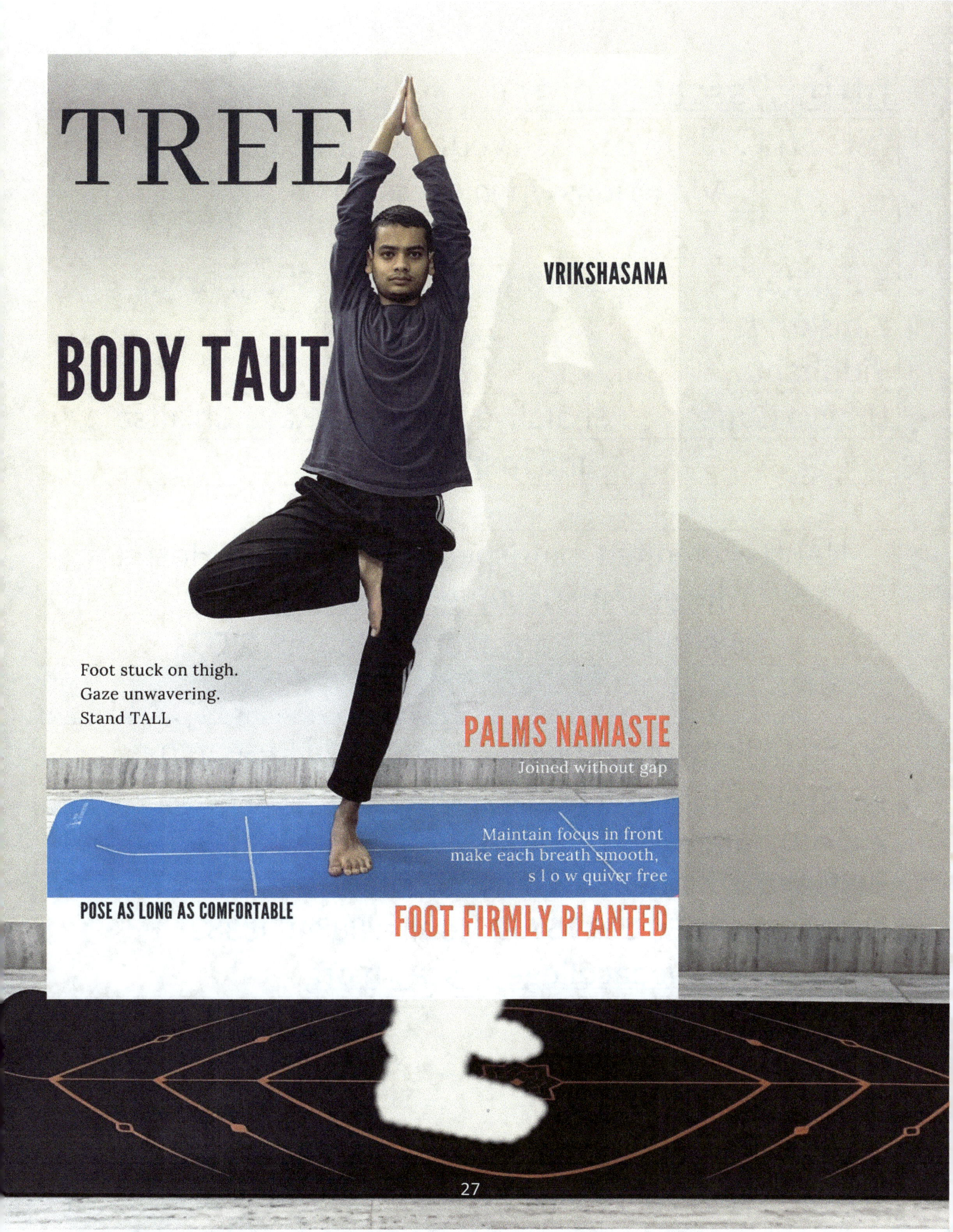
TREE
VRIKSHASANA
BODY TAUT
Foot stuck on thigh.
Gaze unwavering.
Stand TALL
PALMS NAMASTE
Joined without gap
Maintain focus in front
make each breath smooth,
s l o w quiver free
POSE AS LONG AS COMFORTABLE
FOOT FIRMLY PLANTED

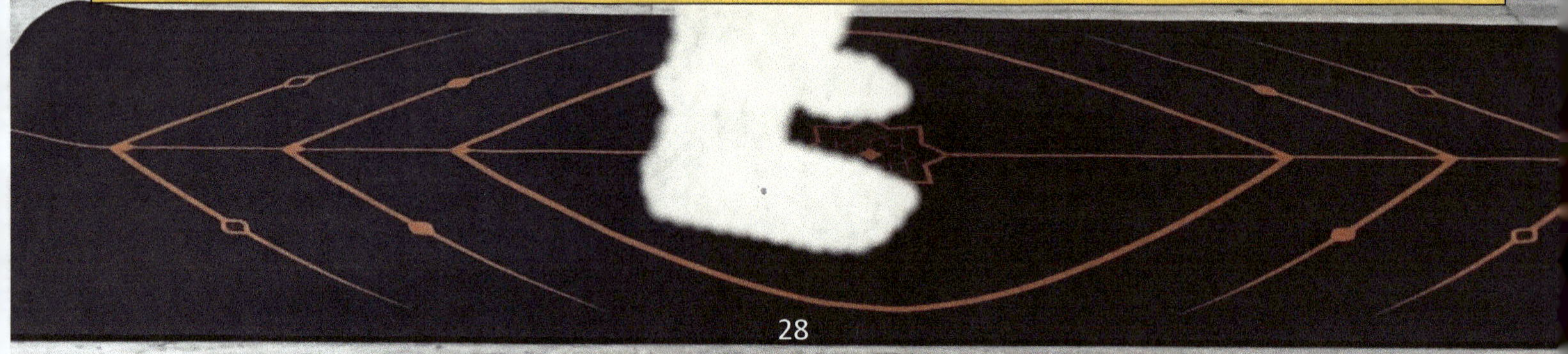

Butterfly – Titli āsana

MIND WHAT'S HAPPENING
Rather light in the head, not so many thoughts.

BODY WHERE IS THE EFFECT
Pelvis, Thighs, Sacrum.

ATTENTION

- On your inner thighs, groin and hips.
- On your chest.
- Focus on the breath and try to breathe without jerks – this brings fluidity in both asana and mind.
- On Swadhisthana and Anahata Chakra –sacral and heart chakras.

BREATH

- Keep breathing naturally in the posture.

SEQUENCE

- Sit comfortably with your legs stretched out in front of you.
- Bending your knees, bring the feet close to the groin and join the soles of your feet.
- Interlock your fingers over the toes and clasp the front part of the foot with your palms; make sure your elbows are close to your body.
- Keep your spine straight, head straight and shoulders relaxed.
- Flap your knees up and down; gently try to push the knees down every time.
- Close your eyes and pick up speed.
- To come out of the posture, unclasp your hands and push your knees up so that the feet are flat on the floor and the knees are joined together. Put your arms around the knees, take your head close to the knees and give yourself a squeezy hug; squeeze especially your thighs and calves. Then, stretch the legs.

COUNTER POSE = Stretch the legs and bring the knees close to the chest and squeeze the thighs together, and again stretch the legs. This can be repeated a few times to realign all the muscles of the legs.

7 Steps 7 Minutes

7 ASPECTS

Day 1
Hold an Asana for 7 Minutes.

Day 2
Do Ujjayi breath for 7 Minutes.

Day 3
Do a Short Meditation.

BUTTERFLY

BODY LIMP

TITLI ASANA

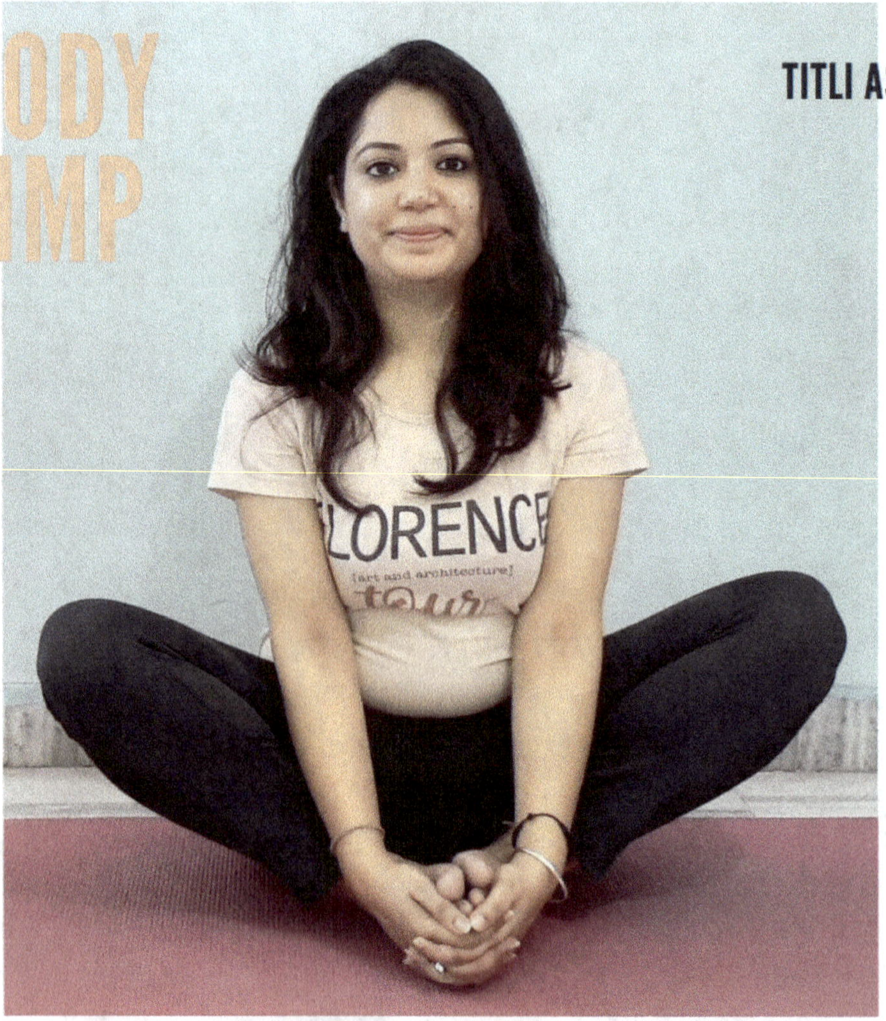

FLAP THE BUTTS MIMIC A BUTTERFLY

FLY CHEERFULLY FOR 2 MINUTES

BUTTERFLY

BODY LIMP

TITLI ASANA

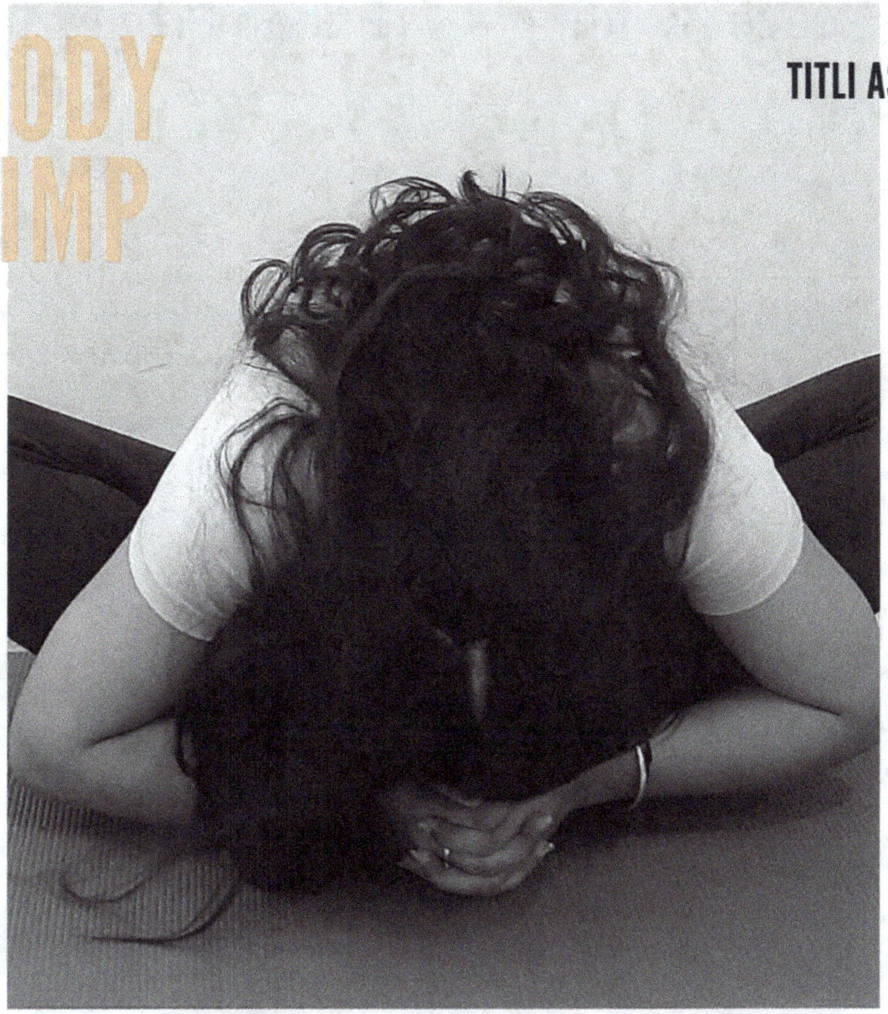

AFTER BUTTERFLYING BOW DOWN

TOUCH THE GROUND

BOW FOR FEW SECONDS

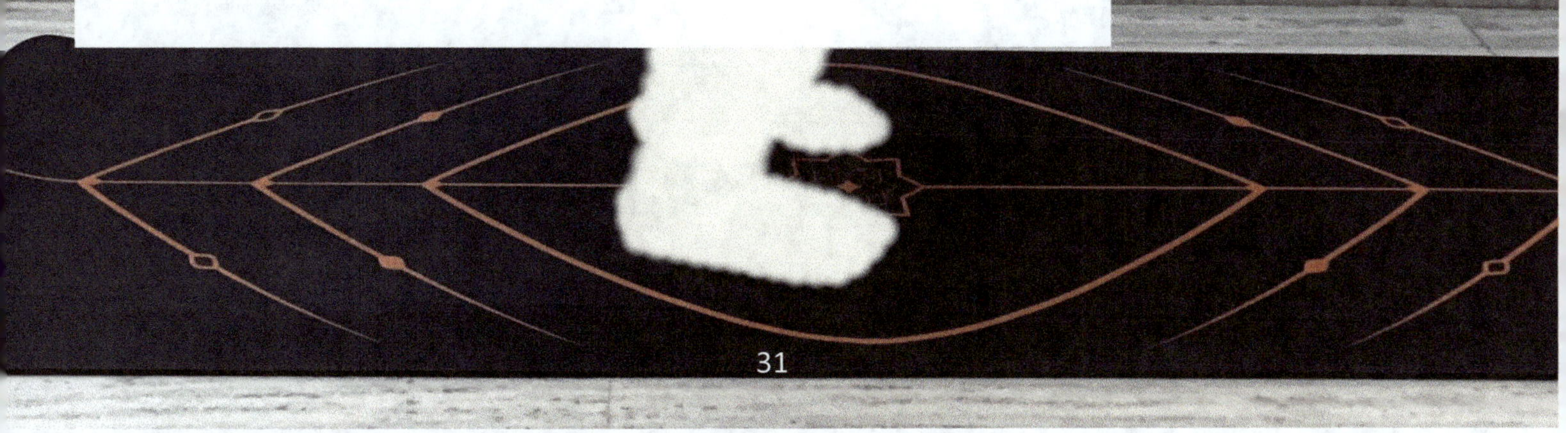

https://www.iahv.org/

International Association for Human Values		
Programs for Institutions, Governments, Planet Earth		
Disaster and Trauma Relief	Peace Building	Prison Program
SKY Campus	Green Pocket Forests	Initiatives for Children
and many others		
Worldwide Presence		

IAHV America
2401, 15th Street NW,
Washington, DC 20009, USA
Landline: +1 202 250 3405
Email ID: info@iahv.org

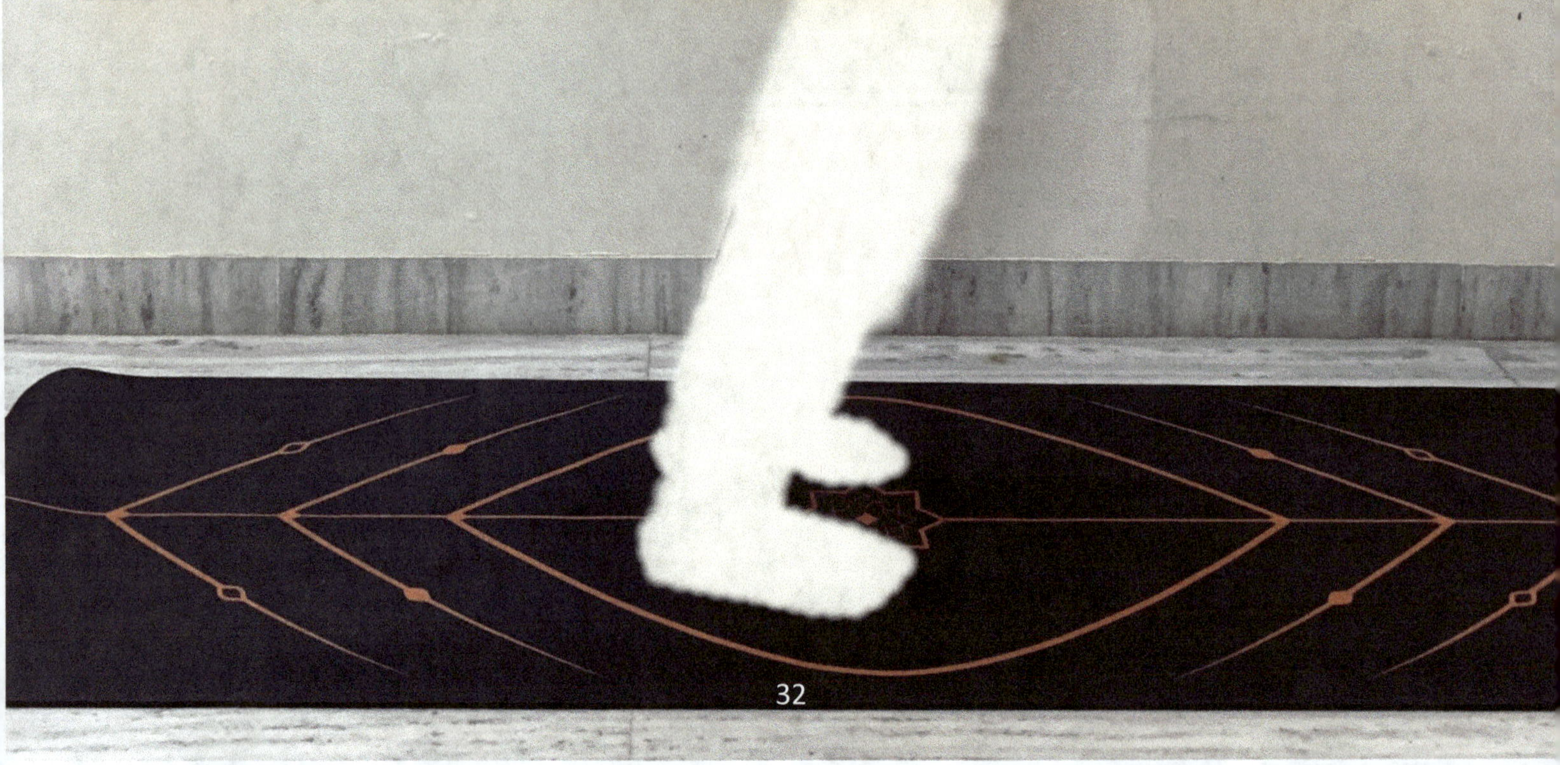

Headstand - Shirsāsana

MIND WHAT'S HAPPENING
Rather light in the head, not so many thoughts.

BODY WHERE IS THE EFFECT
All systems of the body. Neck, Eyes.

ATTENTION
On the third eye.

BREATH
Bit laborious.

SEQUENCE

- Sit in Vajrasana. Do some neck rotation with eyes closed.
- Go forward, place forearms on the floor with hands clasped, and elbows near the knees.
- Bring the head to touch the clasped palms firmly.
- Lift the knees off the floor in a triangle pose.
- Slowly walk the feet towards the head and make the back vertical.
- Bend the legs and press the thighs to the stomach.
- Raise one foot off the floor, then the other, balancing on the head and palms, knees bent.
- Slowly make the legs straight, feet towards the ceiling, limp.
- Hold the posture for a count of 6 Breaths. Breath smoothly.
- When ready to release, Breathe OUT, bend the knees and bring the legs down.

Adjust yourself, realign your muscles, then relax in shavasana.

COUNTER POSE = Neck movements

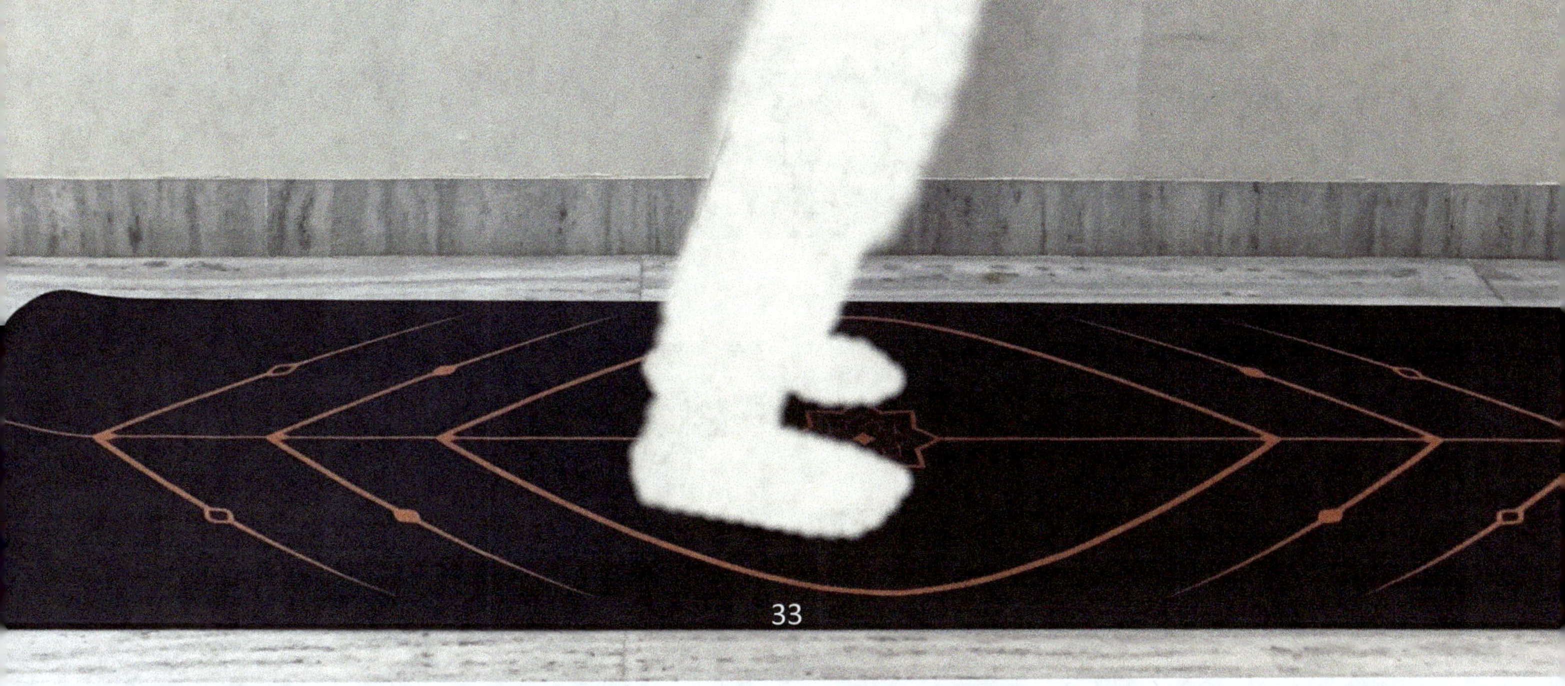

HEADSTAND

ADVANCED

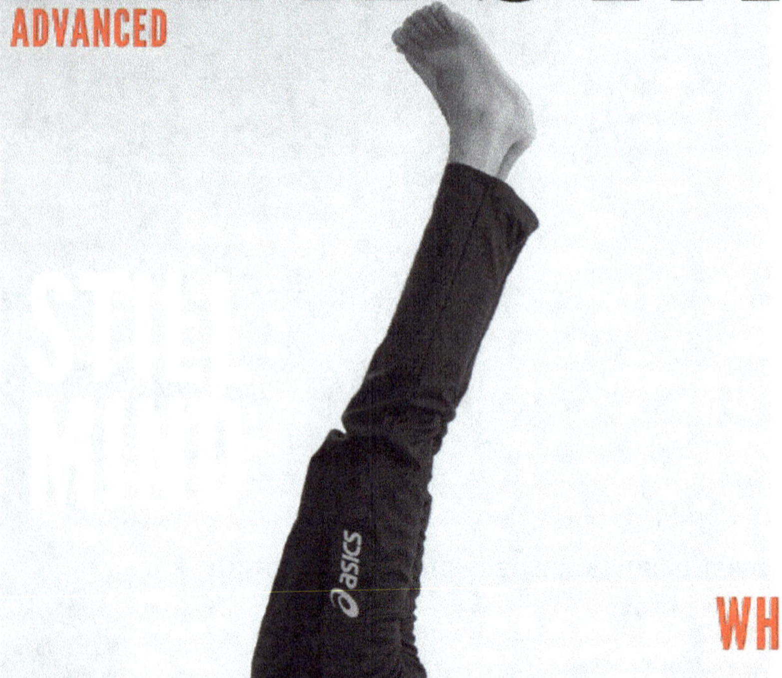

SHIRSHASANA

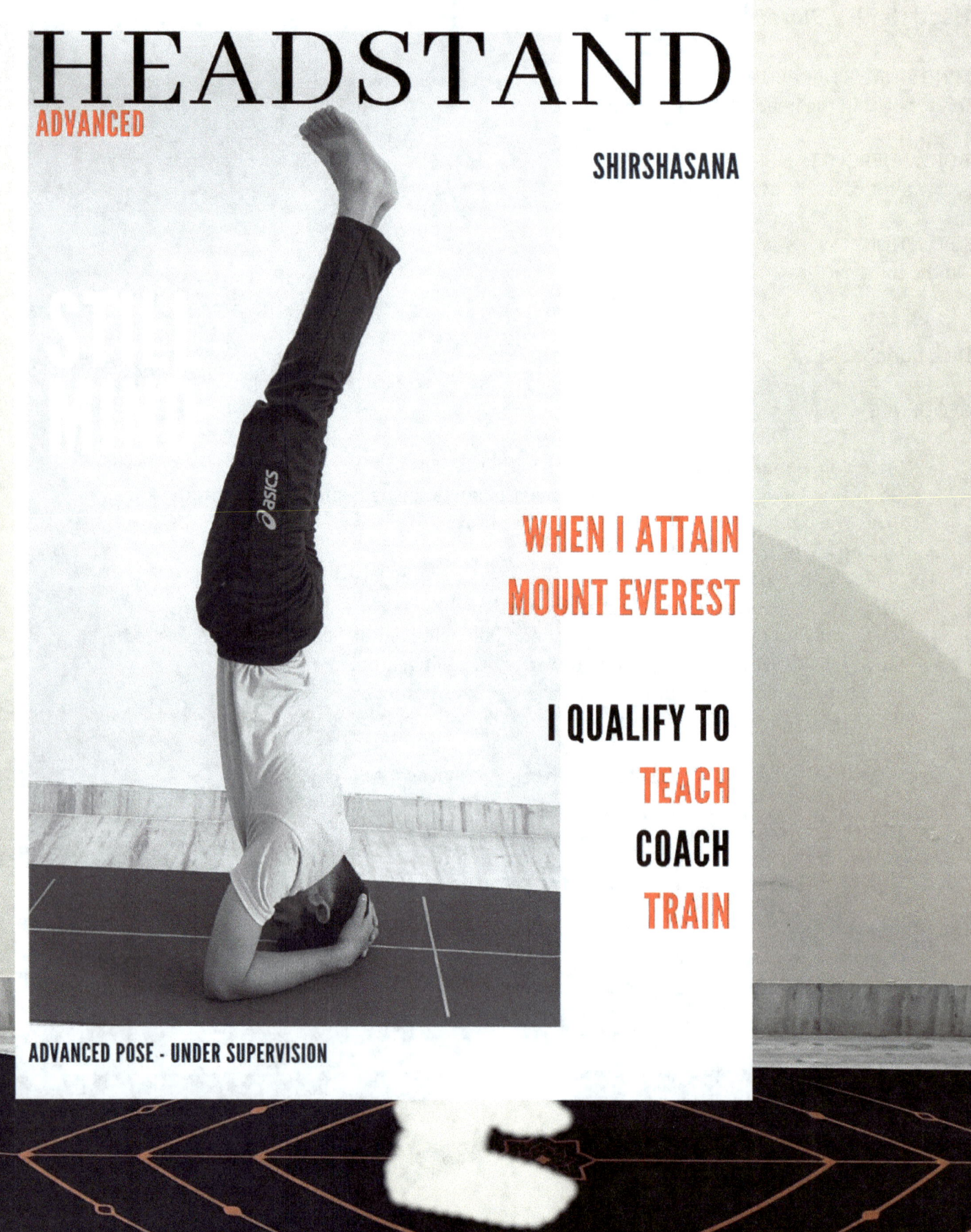

WHEN I ATTAIN
MOUNT EVEREST

I QUALIFY TO
TEACH
COACH
TRAIN

ADVANCED POSE - UNDER SUPERVISION

HEADSTAND

SHIRSHASANA

PINNACLE HUMBLED

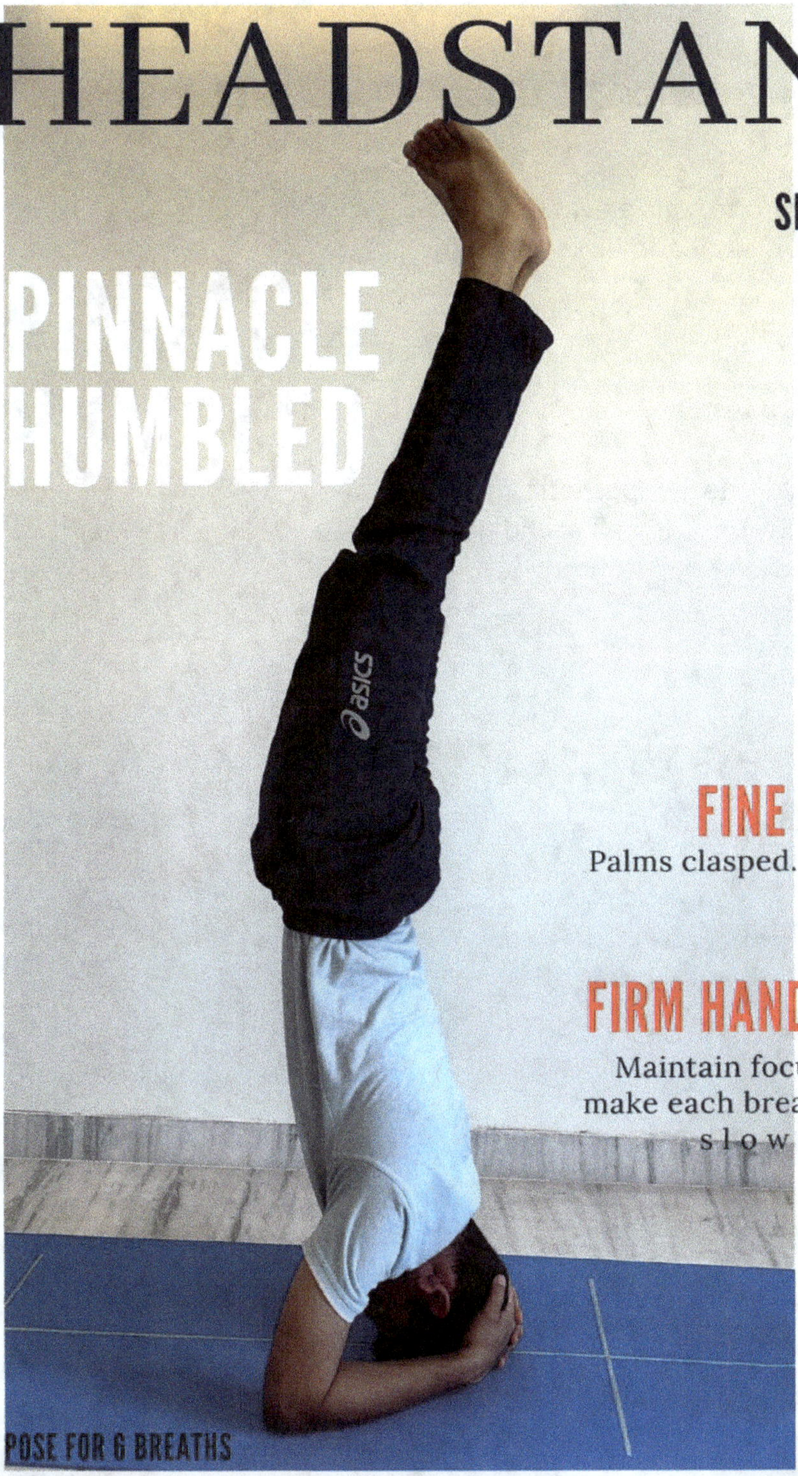

FINE BALANCE

Palms clasped. Head at ease

FIRM HANDS ARMS

Maintain focus on eyes,
make each breath smooth
s l o w quiver-free

POSE FOR 6 BREATHS

One may use the wall for support to practice initially.

Relaxation Poses

After each set of 20 to 40 minutes of asana practice, we must spend some moments in deep relaxation.

Yoga is a process whereby at each moment one feels elevated and energized, and this is made possible by sufficient and timely relaxation.

Opposite Values are Complementary in Nature.

After a session of intense activity, take deep rest.

This helps in tuning and proper balancing of the Sympathetic and Parasympathetic Nervous Systems, thereby ensuring all round health.

7 Steps 7 Minutes

7 ASPECTS

RELAX Often

- Correctly

else

- Senses become dull.
- Decisions become invalid,
- Failure knocks.

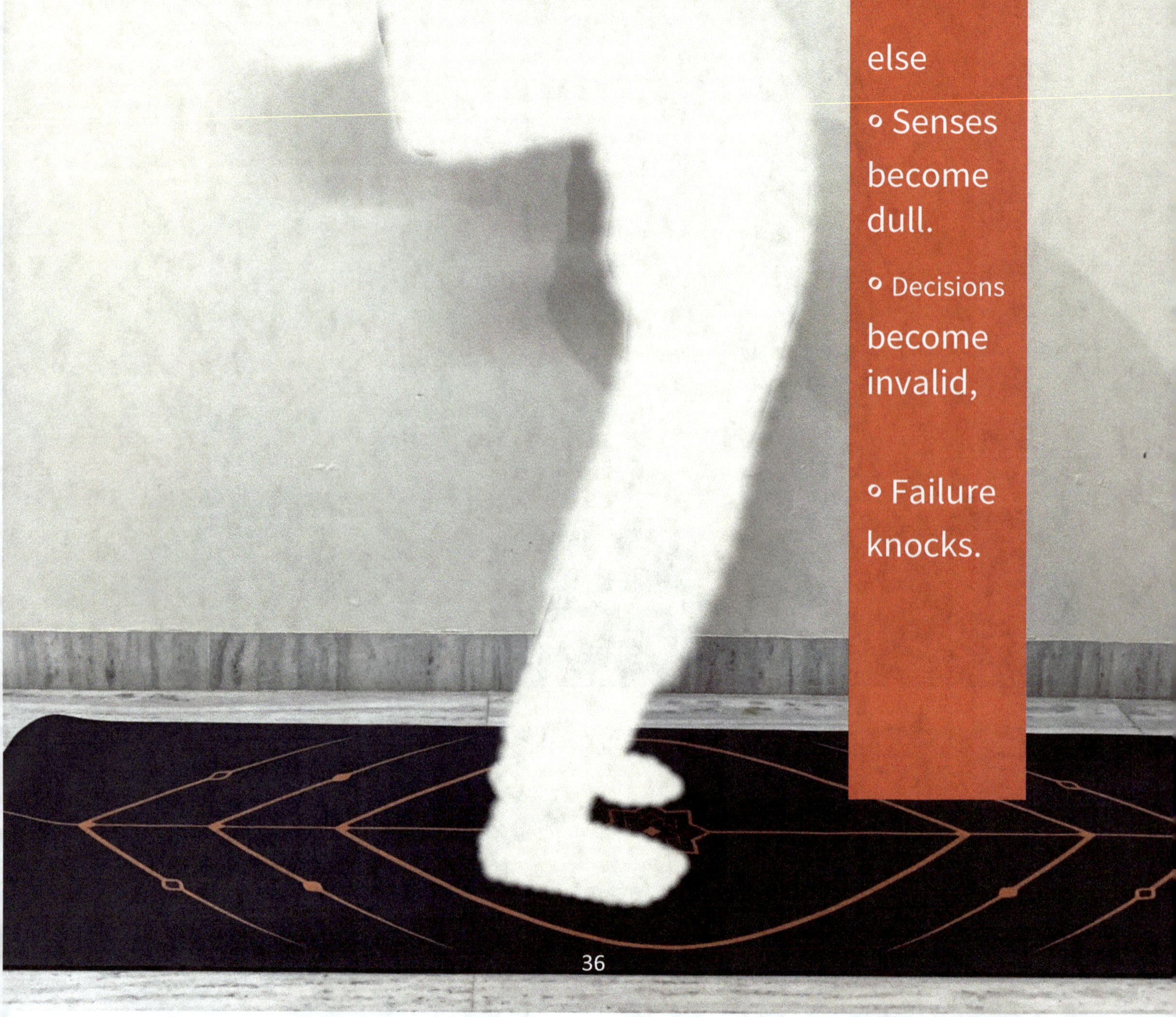

Corpse Pose - Shavāsana

MIND WHAT'S HAPPENING
Rather light in the head, deep rest.

BODY WHERE IS THE EFFECT
Circulatory System, Central Nervous System.

ATTENTION
Let go and space out.

BREATH
Smooth and Natural breathing.

SEQUENCE

- Lie down SUPINE on the back.
- Feet wide apart, toes pointing outward. Knees straight.
- Keep the arms limp near the sides of the body.
- Palms open to the sky.
- Relax for as long as comfortable.

Adjust yourself, realign your muscles, roll over to right side.

COUNTER POSE = Sit up and start doing your duties

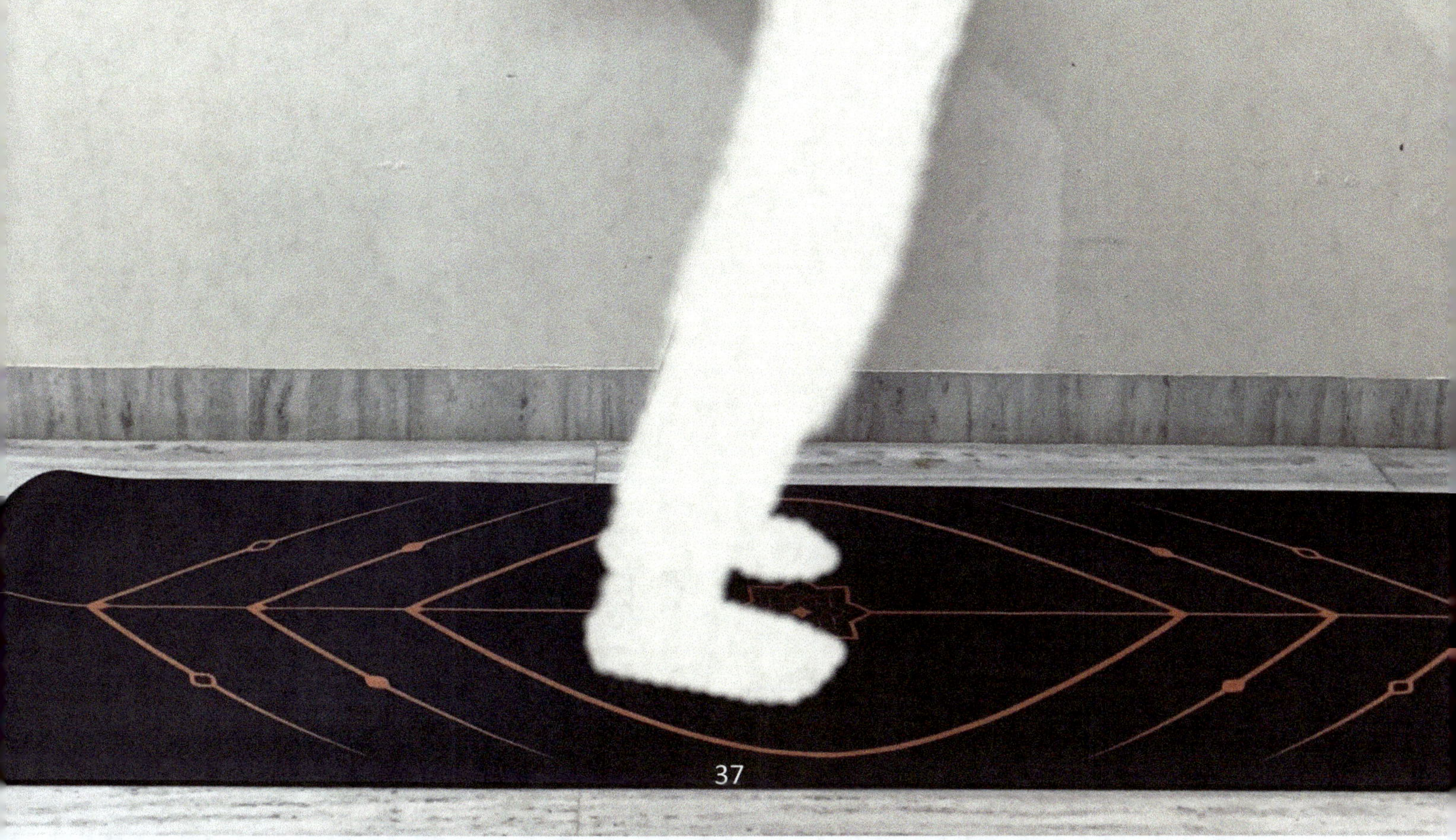

CORPSE

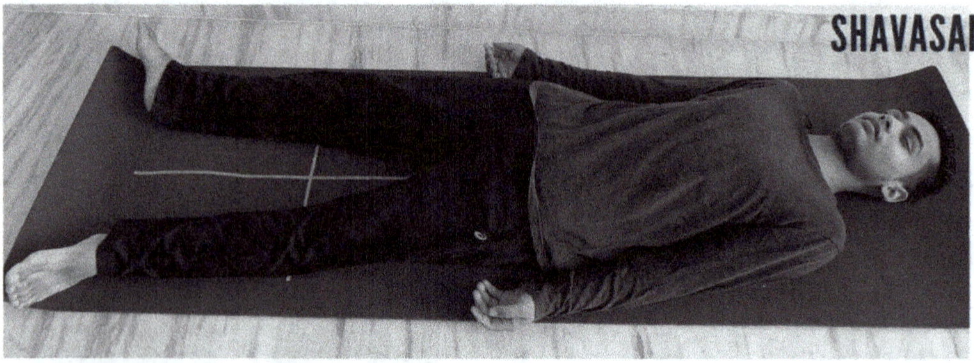

SHAVASANA

BODY DROPS MIND ELEVATES

CONSCIOUSNESS

EXPANDS

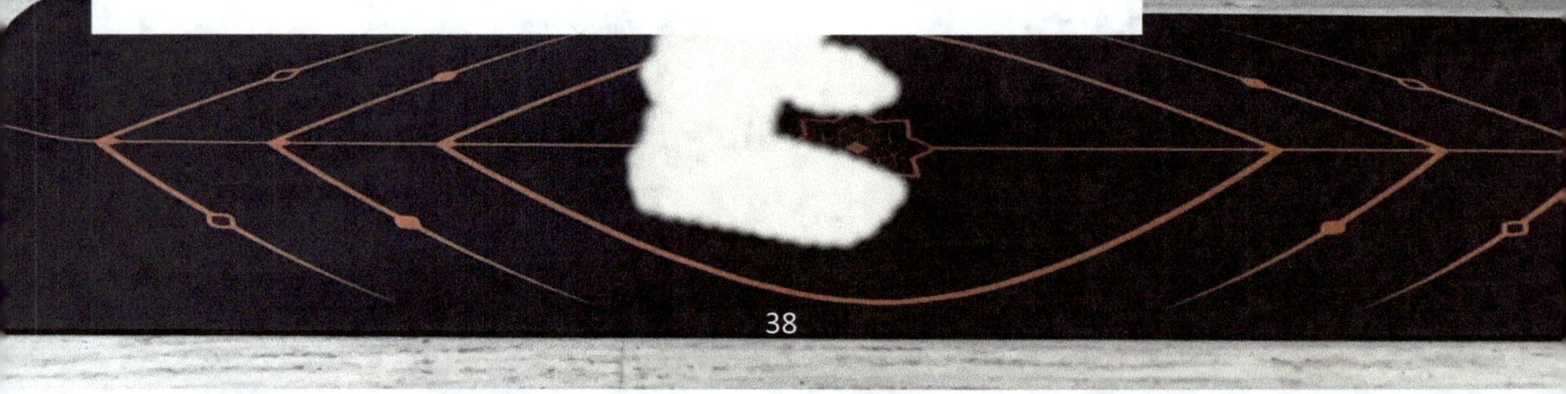

CORPSE

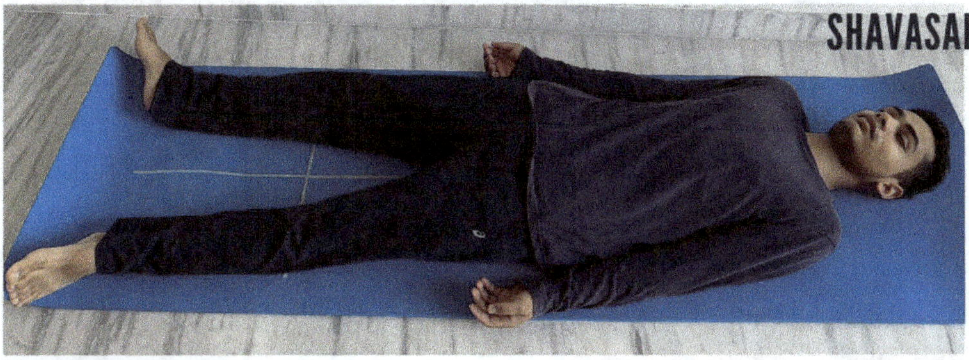

SHAVASANA

BODY LIMP

LEGS APART FEET OUT

Neck loose. Face Relaxed.
Delicate sleep

ARMS NEAR BODY

Let go the focus, make
each breath smooth s l o w
quiver-free

POSE AS LONG AS COMFORTABLE

Crocodile - Makarāsana

MIND WHAT'S HAPPENING
Rather light in the head, deep rest.

BODY WHERE IS THE EFFECT
Lower back, lumbar, pelvis, and hips.

ATTENTION
Let go and space out.

BREATH
Smooth and Natural breathing.

SEQUENCE

- Lie down PRONE on the stomach.
- Feet wide apart, toes pointing outward. Knees straight.
- Keep one palm over the other facing down and rest the forehead on the palms.
- Entire body is loose and at a slight angle.
- Relax for as long as comfortable.

Adjust yourself, realign your muscles, roll over to shavasana.

COUNTER POSE = Shavasana

7 Steps 7 Minutes

7 ASPECTS

RELAXati-on does magic to the Body.

- Even the mind becomes charged and cheerful.
- Relax for at least 7 minutes.

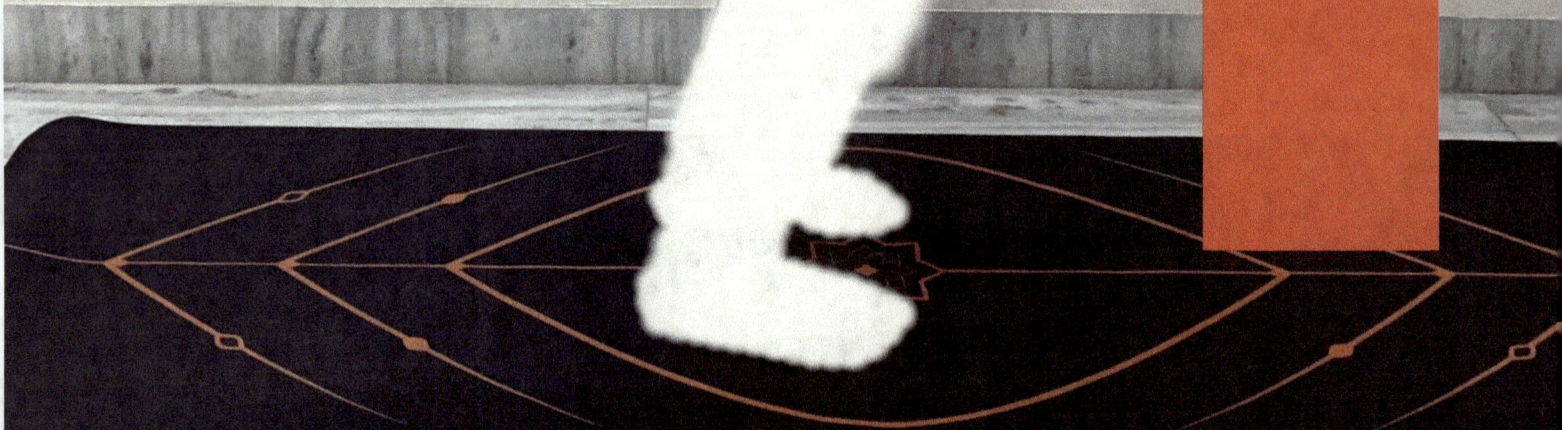

CROCODILE

MAKARASANA

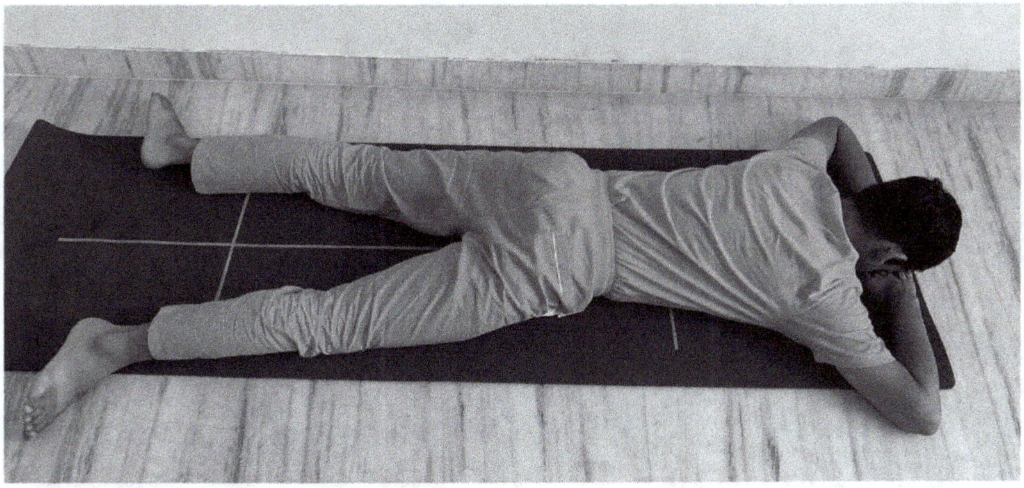

BACK WELL RESTED

I SENSE DEEP PEACE

CROCODILE

MAKARASANA

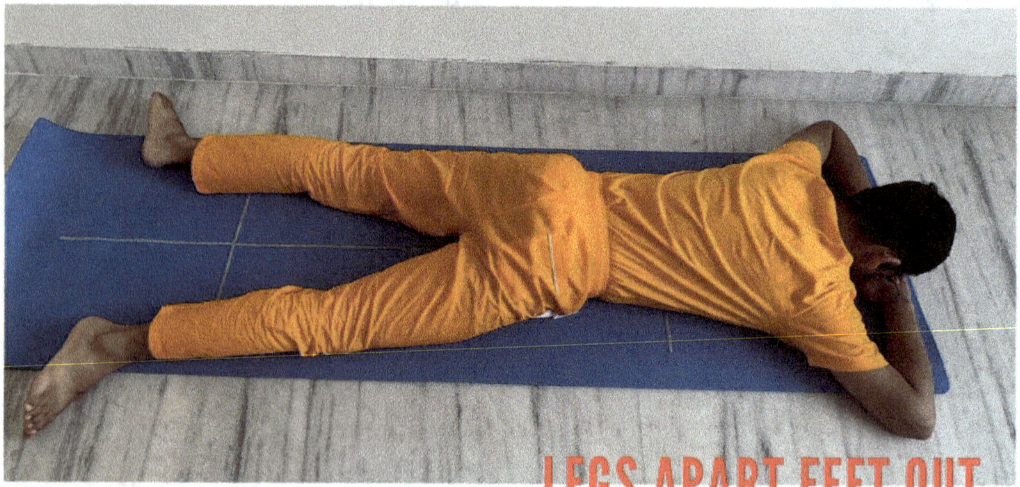

LEGS APART FEET OUT

Neck loose. Face Relaxed.
Delicate sleep

BODY LIMP

HEAD ON PALMS

Let go the focus, make
each breath smooth s l o w
quiver-free

POSE AS LONG AS COMFORTABLE

Prone Vishnu

MIND WHAT'S HAPPENING
Rather light in the head, deep rest.

BODY WHERE IS THE EFFECT
Shoulders, Lower back, abdomen, pelvis, and thigh.

ATTENTION
Let go and space out.

BREATH
Smooth and Natural breathing.

SEQUENCE

- Lie down PRONE on the stomach.
- Feet together. Knees straight.
- Bend the Right leg and keep it limp.
- Right Arms by the face, Left Hand near the Head, palms facing down, fingers open.
- Relax for as long as comfortable.

Adjust yourself, realign your muscles, roll over to shavasana.

Can do with other leg on another occasion.

COUNTER POSE = Shavasana

7 Steps 7 Minutes

7 ASPECTS

At times

- One feels one shall miss an import-ant meeting.
- Or a deadline, and work oneself to death in the process!

PRONE

VISHNU

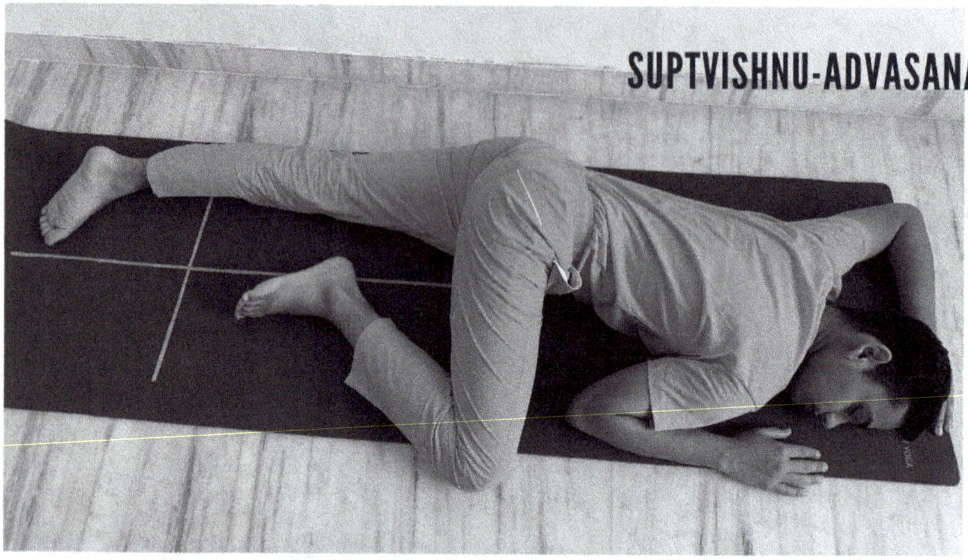

SUPTVISHNU-ADVASANA

UMM MOST RELAXING

RELAX LET GO TO UNLEASH CREATIVITY

PRONE

VISHNU

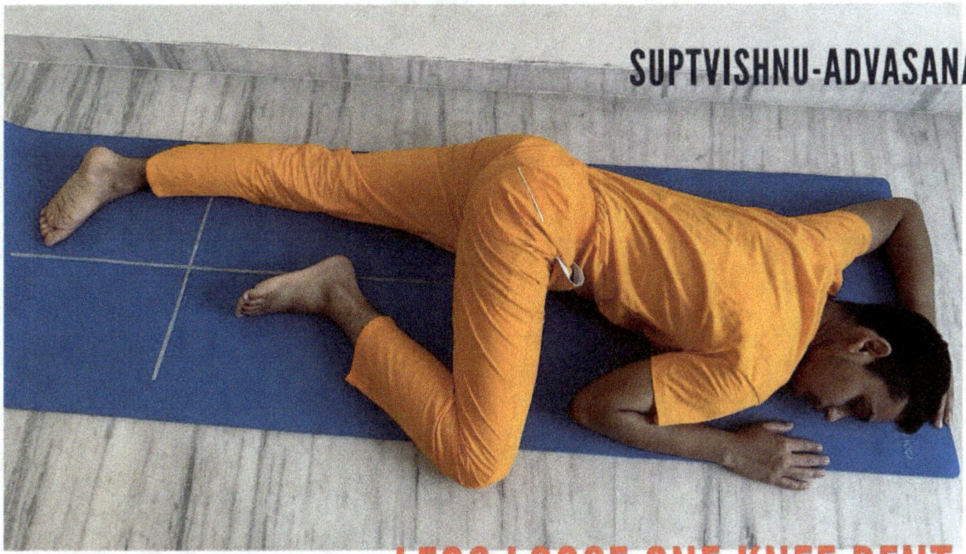

SUPTVISHNU-ADVASANA

BODY LIMP

LEGS LOOSE ONE KNEE BENT

Neck loose. Face Relaxed.
Delicate sleep

PALMS OPEN TO FLOOR

Let go the focus, make
each breath smooth s l o w
quiver-free

POSE AS LONG AS COMFORTABLE

https://worldforumforartandculture.com

World Forum for Art and Culture

An Online Initiative for Music and Dance Learning

Learn Teach Collaborate Perform

Artist Circle	Kala Swadhyaya	Kala Shaala
Dance	Vocal	Instrumental
Folk	Theatre	Literature

Email ID: info@wfac.in

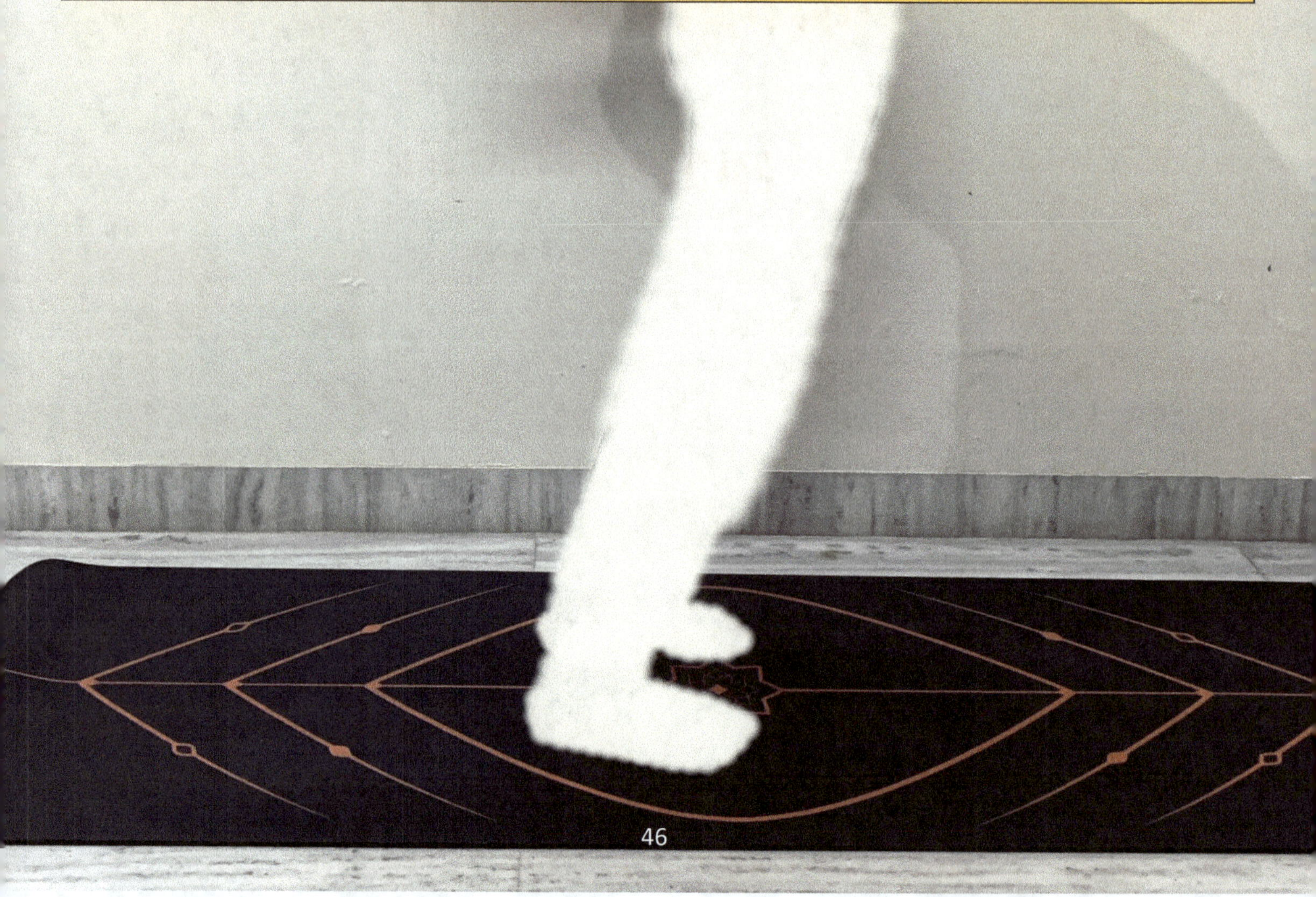

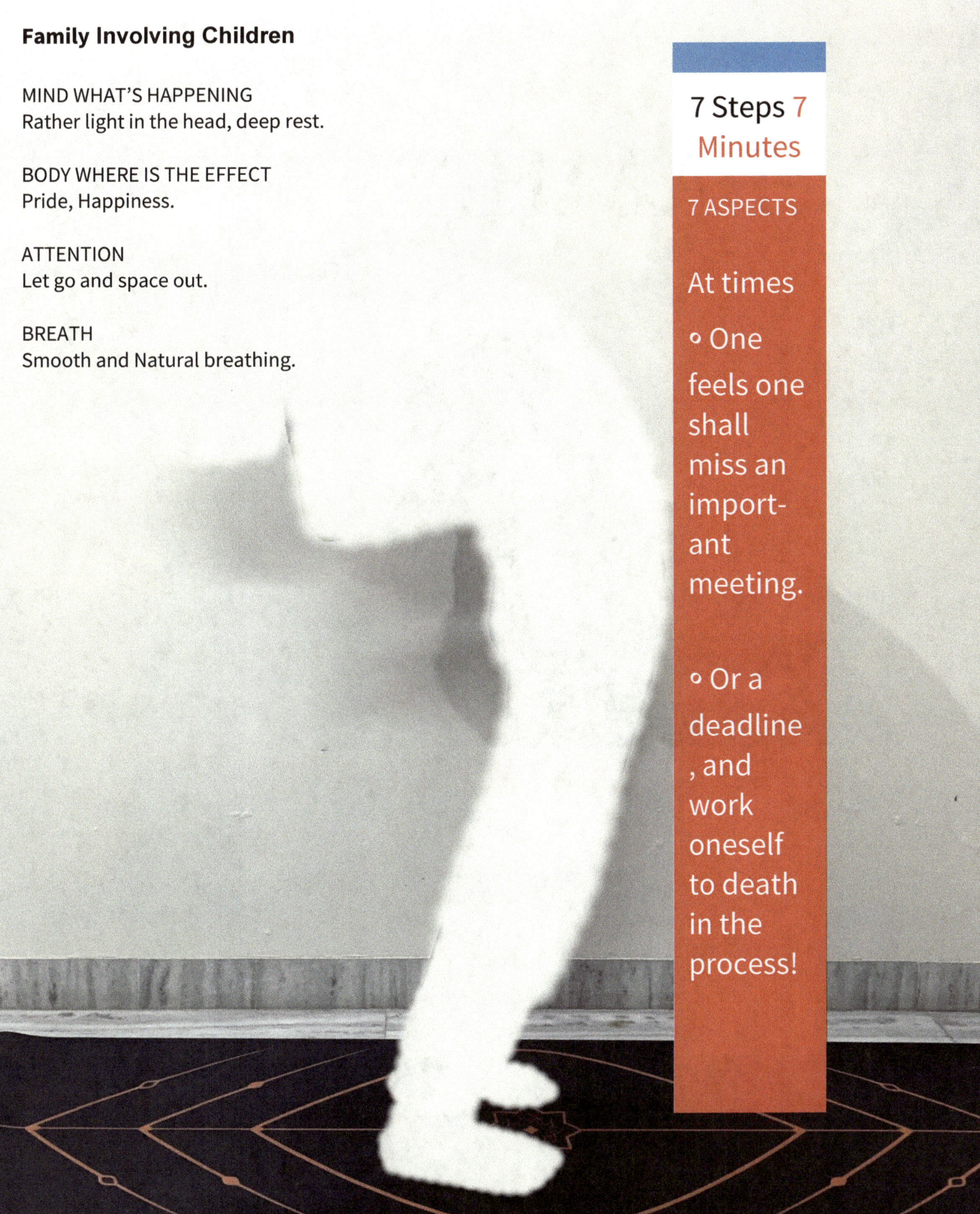

Family Involving Children

MIND WHAT'S HAPPENING
Rather light in the head, deep rest.

BODY WHERE IS THE EFFECT
Pride, Happiness.

ATTENTION
Let go and space out.

BREATH
Smooth and Natural breathing.

7 Steps 7 Minutes

7 ASPECTS

At times

- One feels one shall miss an important meeting.
- Or a deadline, and work oneself to death in the process!

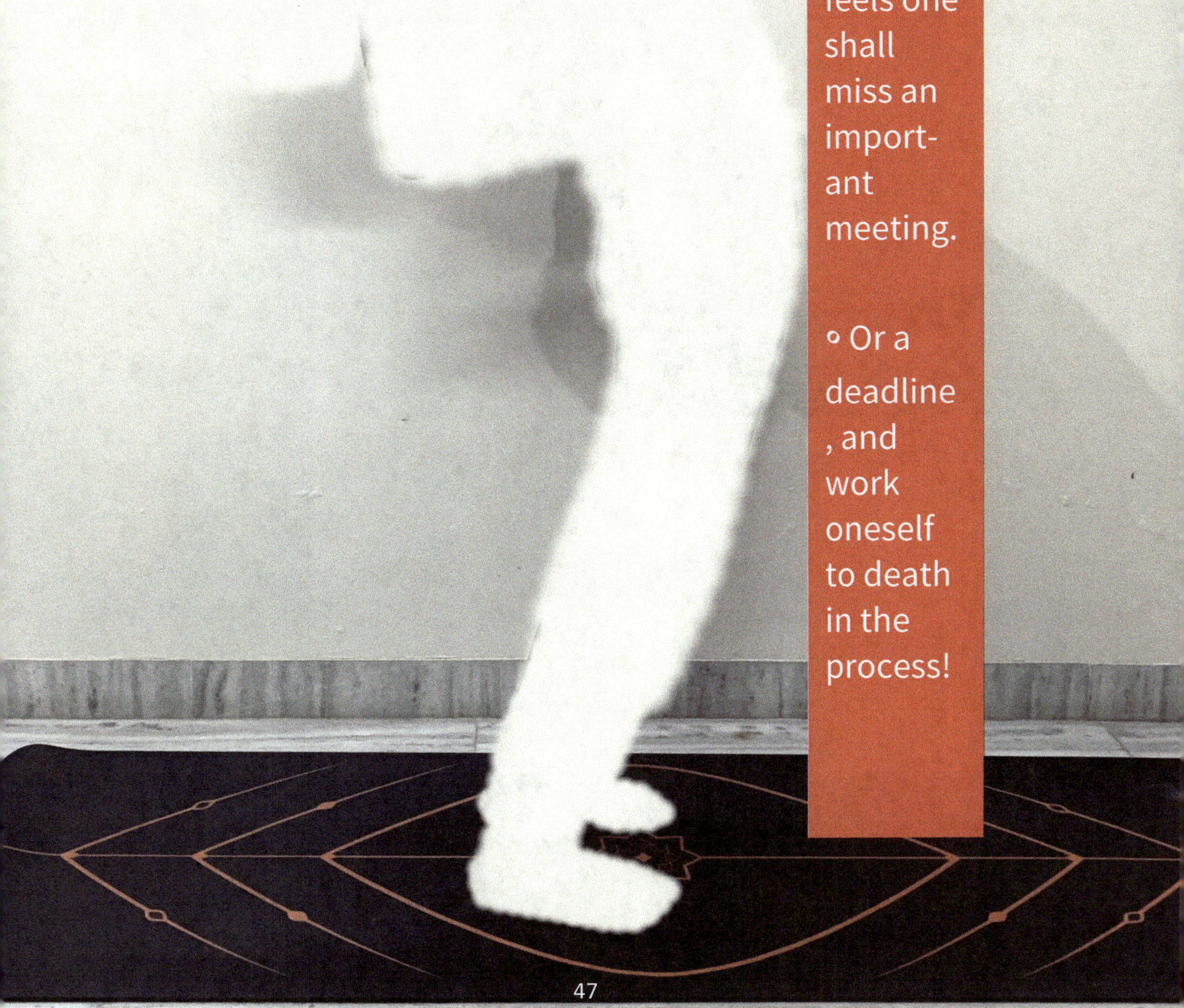

FAMILY

TOGETHER

HOLD STEADY

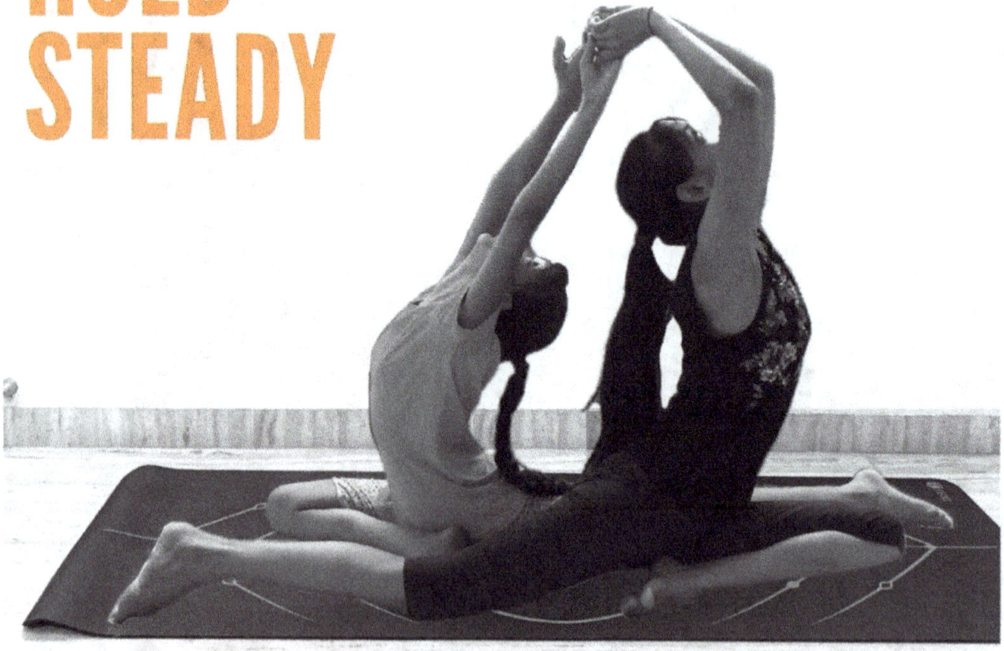

CHILDREN ENJOY A GAME, MOM FEELS PROUD

REPEAT WITH LEGS REVERSED

FAMILY

WE CAN

TOGETHER

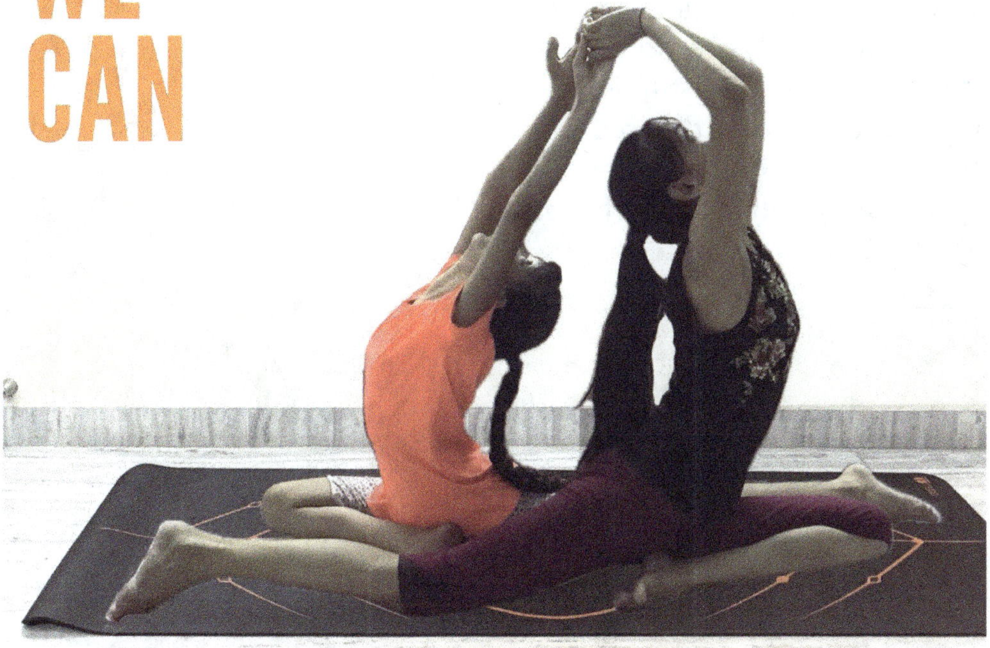

ENCOURAGE YOUNG CHILDREN AT EARLY AGE

Plan in Tandem. Go about it slowly, there's no rush

POSE FOR 20 SECONDS

PATANJALI YOGA SUTRA

तपः–स्वाध्याय–ईश्वरप्रणिधानानि क्रिया–योगः । २.१

tapaḥsvādhyāyeśvarapraṇidhānāni kriyāyogaḥ II 2.1 II

2.1 Tapas, Svadhyaya and Ishvarpranidhana are directives for Yoga

Sadhana for the seeker constitutes of

- tapaḥ = going willfully through discipline and practice, having forbearance.
- svādhyāya = self-study, devoting enough time and priority to personal sadhana, study of scripture and correct dinacharya that suits one's constitution.
- īśvarapraṇidhāna = total surrender to the Lord, acknowledging the presence of a higher power, acknowledging the support of nature and its forces, being devoted to the Master

To Summarize

Yogasana practice is all about

- Posture and Balance
- Strength and Flexibility
- Flow and Rhythm
- Timing and Rest
- Silence and Stillness

Asana practice enhances the mood and delivers on many fronts, and that makes life worthwhile.

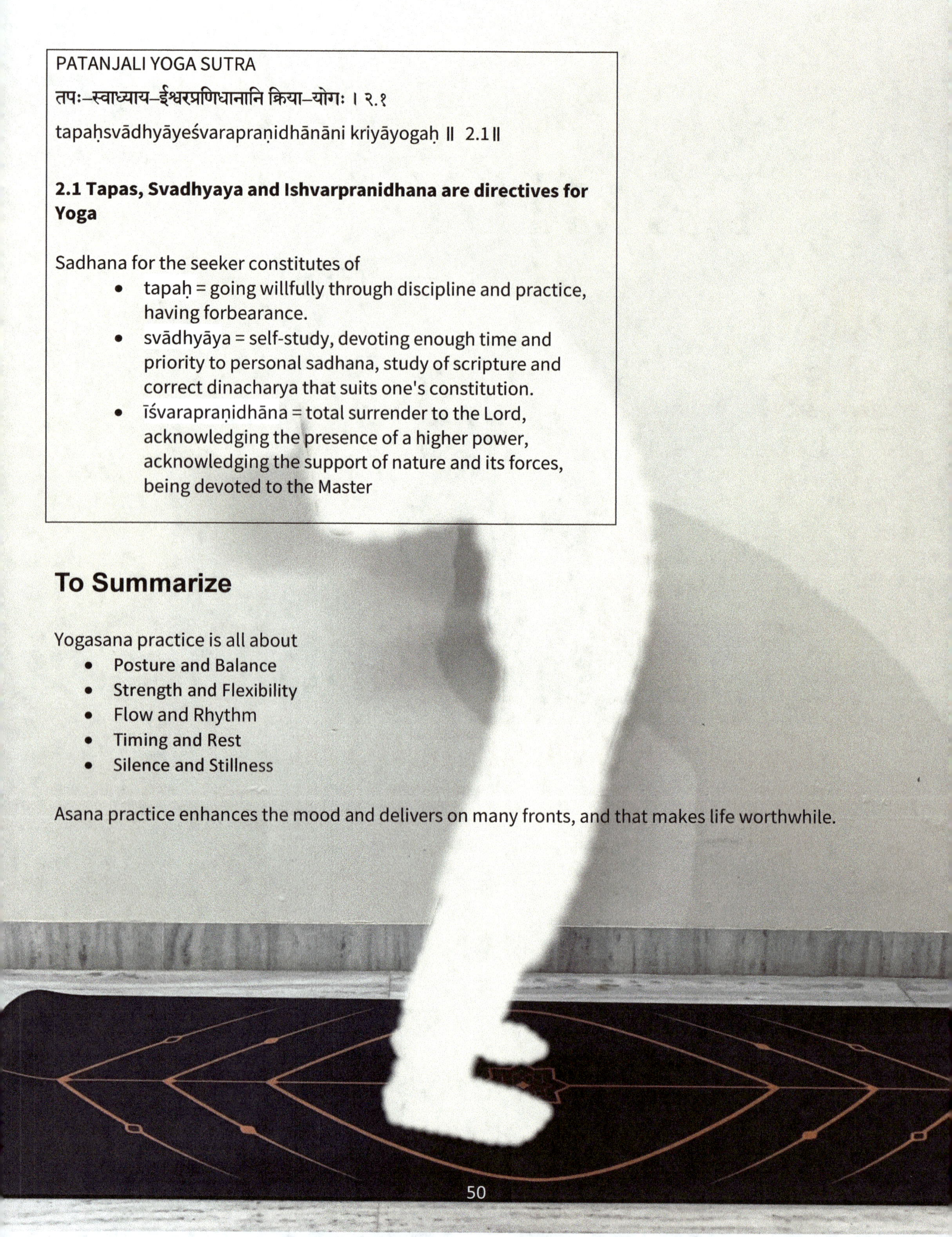

4 Good Bath

Wearing fresh clean clothes will bring the smile easily.

Bathing involves

- using quality soap and reaching to all areas of the skin
- using hair shampoo twice a week
- proper oiling of the joints prior to bath
- oiling the navel and the nostrils well
- oil pulling using virgin coconut oil
- eyes cleaning using triphala water
- using a pumice stone to remove dead skin
- preventing dandruff or taking quick action on its occurrence

Bathing elevates the Mood, balances the Doshas, and is a powerful Tonic for the bodyMind complex.

7 Steps 7 Minutes

7 ASPECTS

Bathing is a forgotten Art.

- It was taken very seriously by men of yore.
- A good bath takes at least 7 minutes.

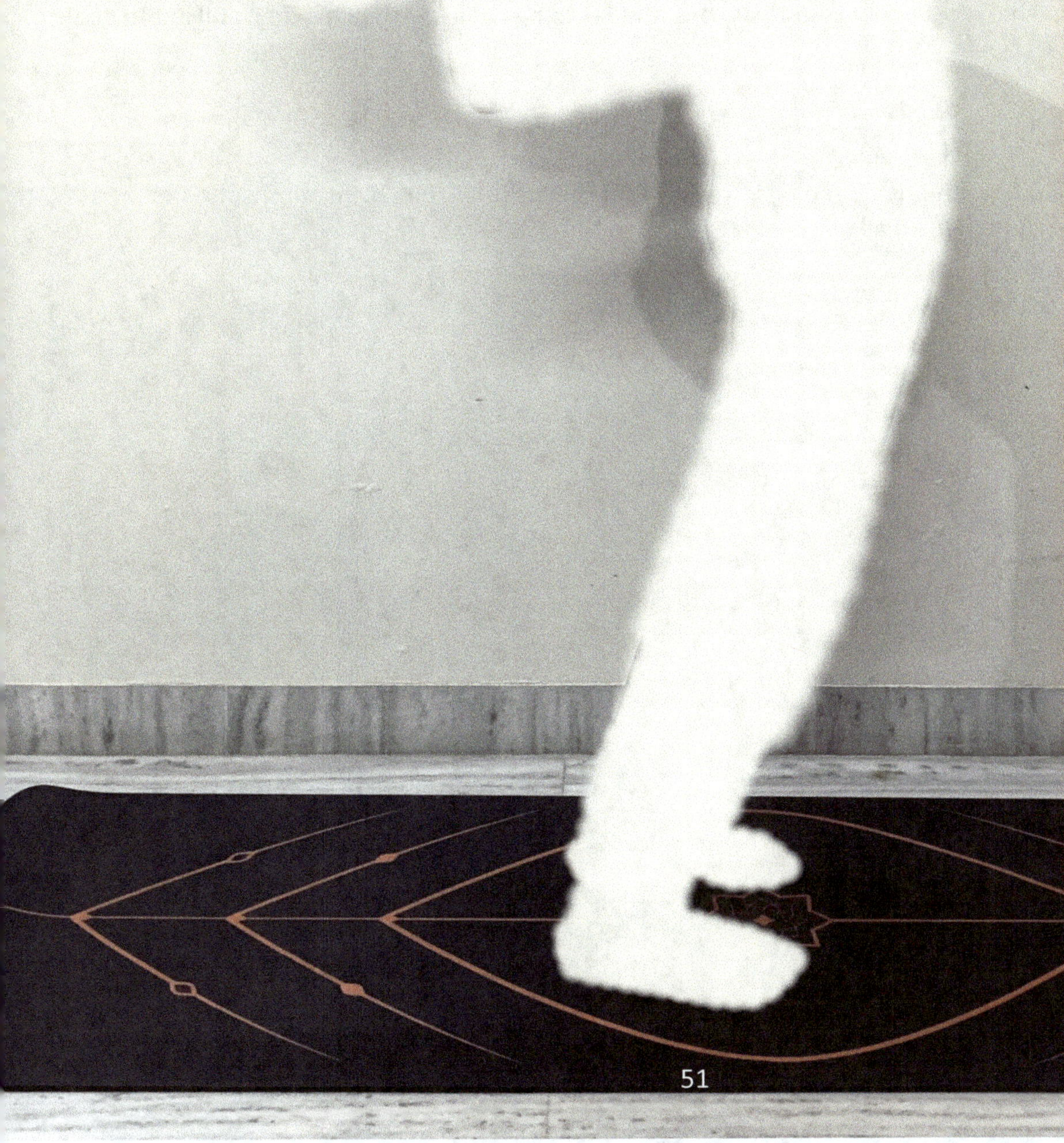

7 Pranayama

Ujjayi Breath

Also known as the Victory Breath, the Ujjayi is the most touted breath in the Yoga tradition, because it quickly brings the senses under control and makes the mind restful and alert.

Breathe with focus on the throat, so that the breath slides along the throat and makes a soft purring sound, just like a snore.

It closely resembles the effort made in sipping a milkshake using a straw.

The sound is akin to the sound from tall floor standing speakers that have been switched on, but have not yet been given audio input.

- It helps very much to do 11 counts of Ujjayi breath first thing while getting up when still in the bed in a half-sleep state.
- Similarly, it is beneficial to do 11 counts of Ujjayi just before dropping to sleep at night.
- In the famous Sudarshan Kriya Happiness Course Program of the Art of Living, this is the first breathing technique that we all learn and have come to relish so much.

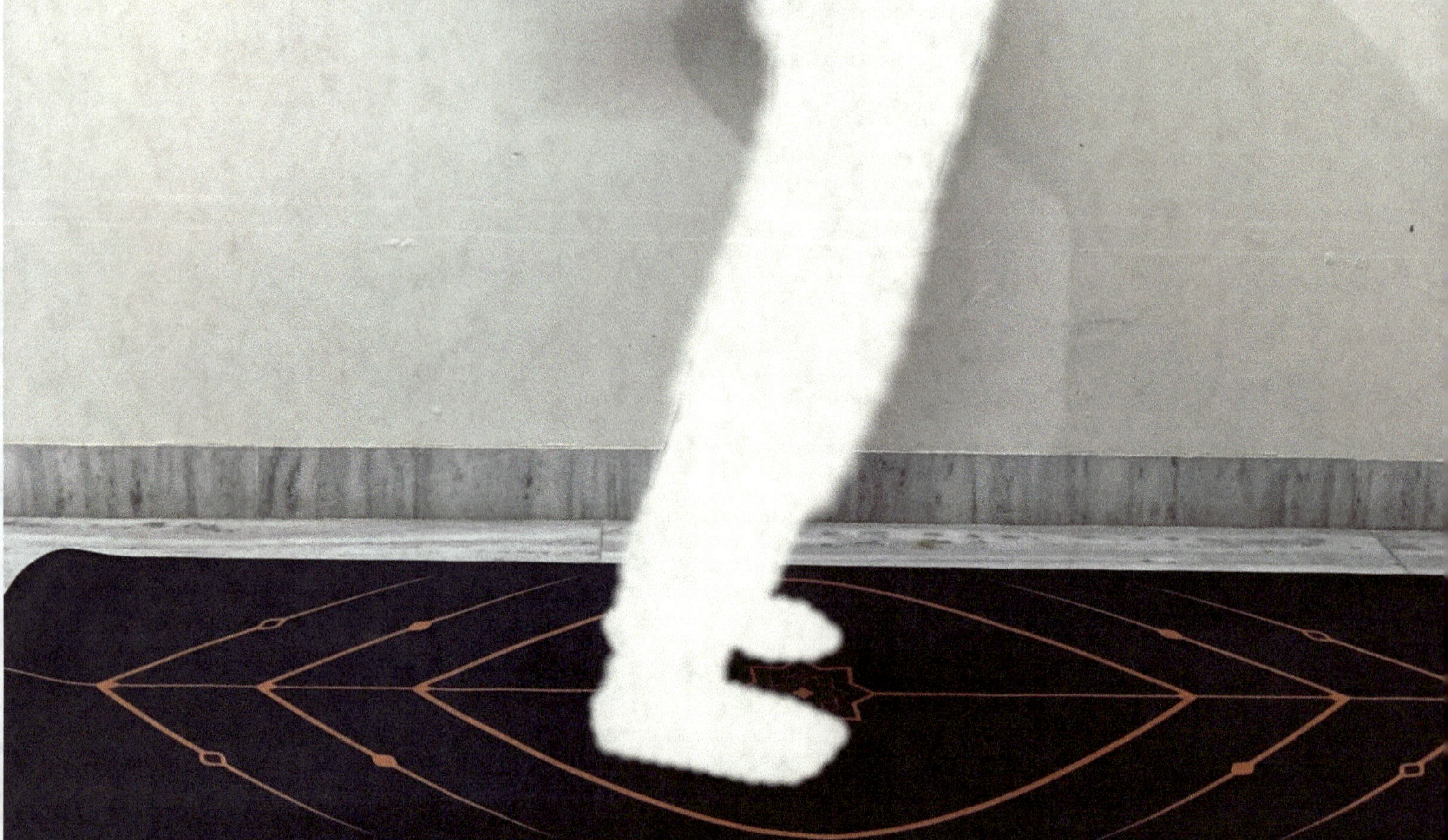

Bhastrikā

MIND WHAT'S HAPPENING
Rather excited and brimming with confidence.

BODY WHERE IS THE EFFECT
All the tissues and cells, the stale air is thrown out from each and every part of the body.

ATTENTION
On the nose.

BREATH
Forceful breathing from the nose with loud sound from the nose.

SEQUENCE

- Sit in Vajrasana.
- Now bring the palms in a fist near the shoulders. Thumb out, nails to the front. Arms near the sides of the chest.
- Body straight and firm.
- With a smile take a normal breath IN and let go.
- Forceful Breathe IN through the nose with a sound, throw both arms UPWARDS (like throwing a basketball) and open the fists. Hover there for a moment.
- As you breathe OUT forcefully through the nose with a loud sound, allow the arms to FALL back to shoulder height and close the hands in a fist, with nails pointing to the front. Allow the elbows to knock the sides of the rib cage while coming DOWN and breathing OUT.
- Continue likewise for 20 breaths. That makes one round.
- When finished, place both palms open to the sky on the knees or in the lap.

Adjust yourself, realign your muscles, keep the eyes closed for few seconds, observe the flow of prana in the body.

COUNTER POSE = Smile Pose

7 Steps 7 Minutes

7 ASPECTS

Ahh Breath!

- Without Trekking or outdoor Sports or ploughing the Soil, one never gets to breathe correctly

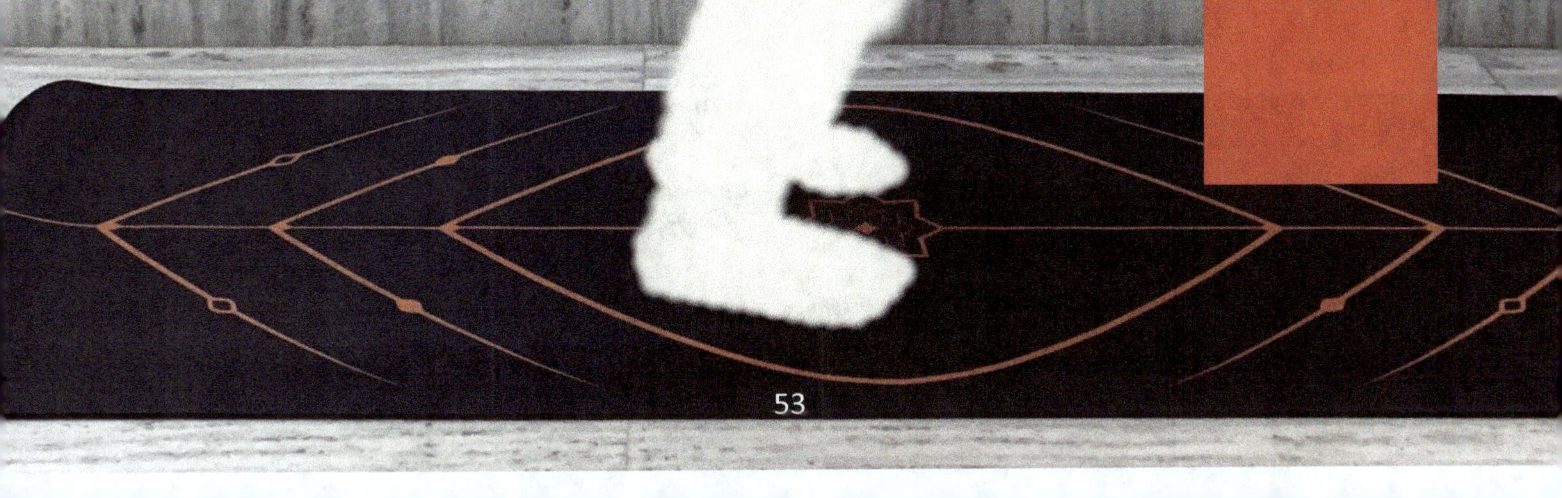

INHALATION POSITION

BELLOWS

BHASTRIKA

BODY FIRM

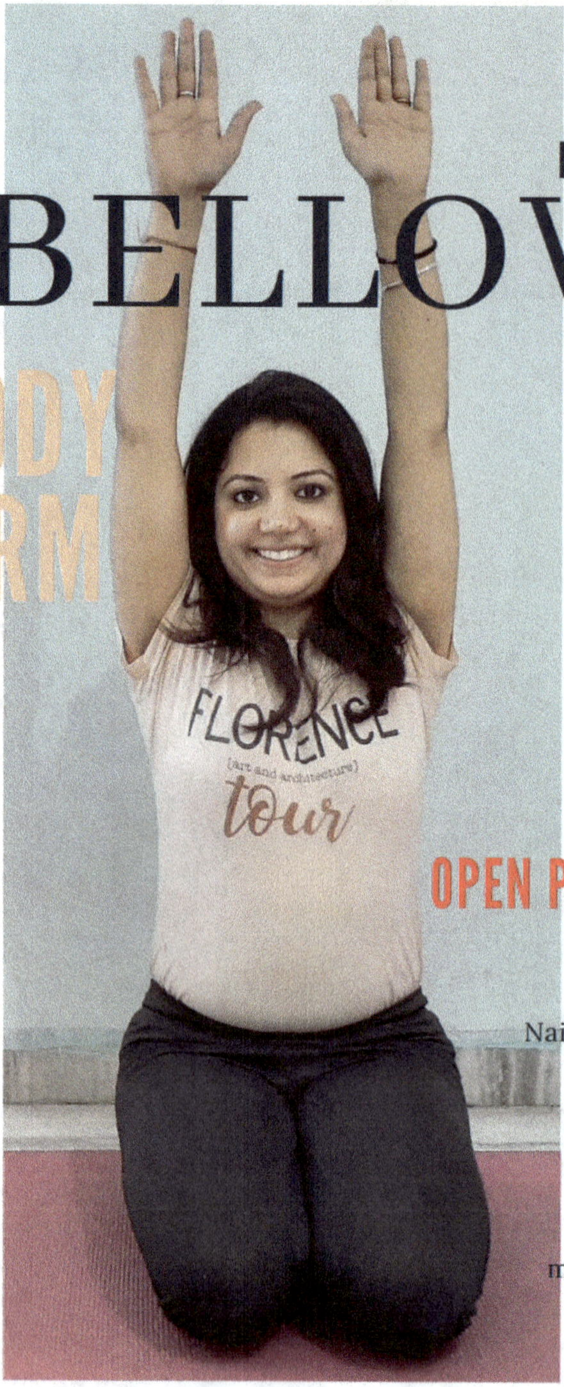

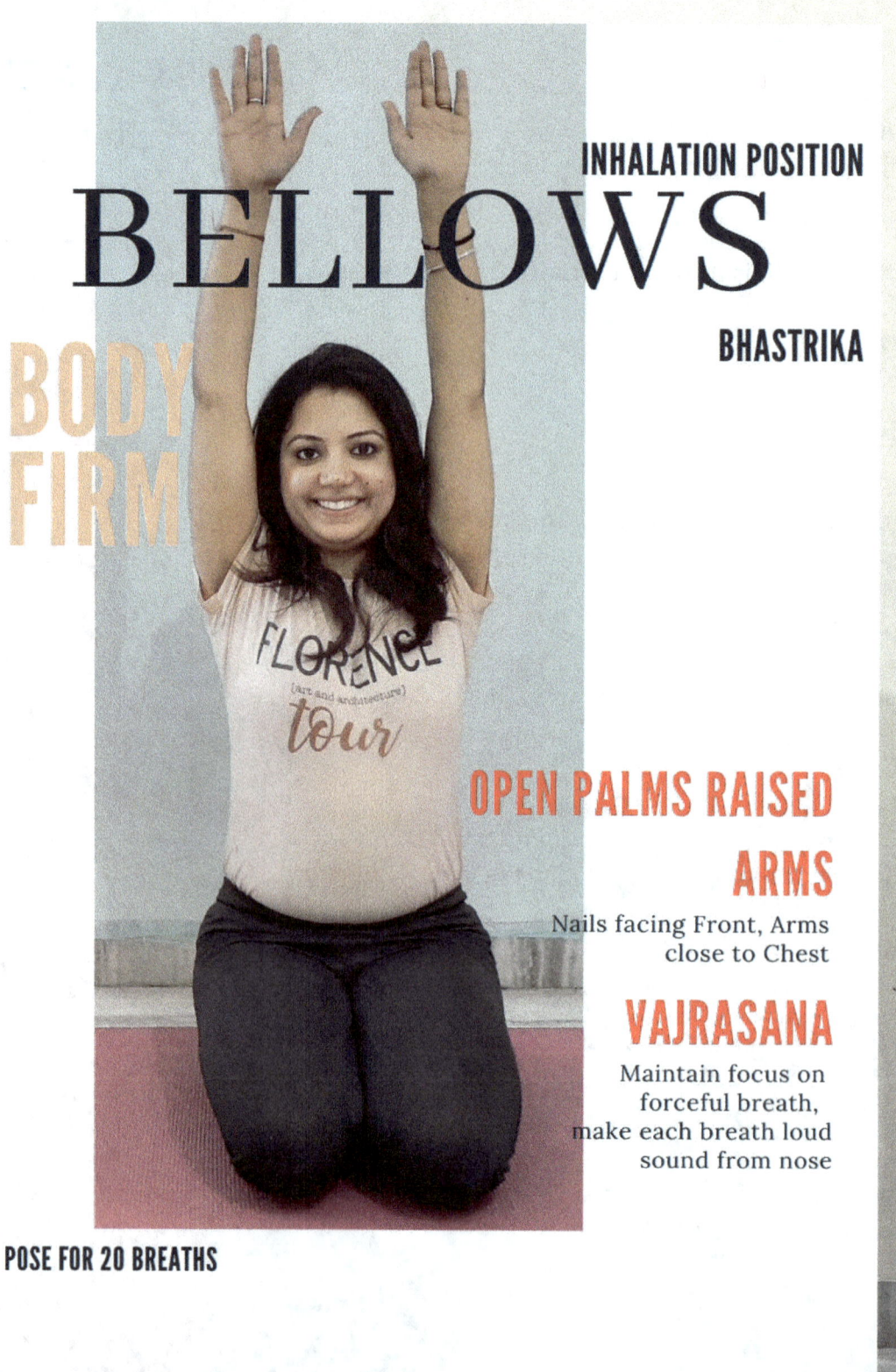

OPEN PALMS RAISED ARMS

Nails facing Front, Arms close to Chest

VAJRASANA

Maintain focus on forceful breath, make each breath loud sound from nose

POSE FOR 20 BREATHS

EXHALATION POSITION

BELLOWS

BHASTRIKA

BODY FIRM

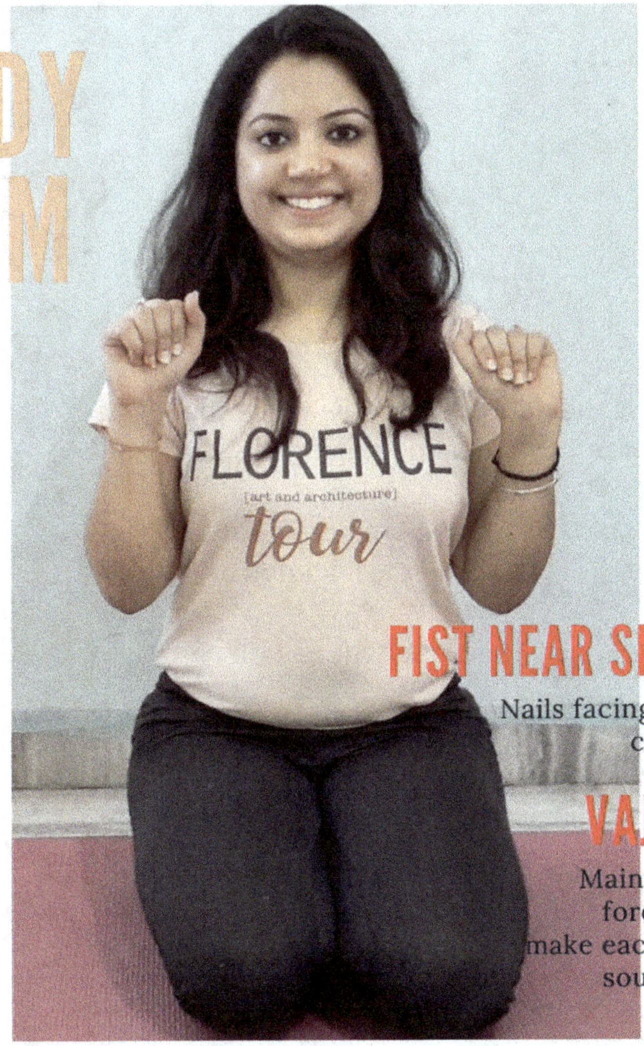

FIST NEAR SHOULDER

Nails facing Front, Arms close to Chest

VAJRASANA

Maintain focus on forceful breath, make each breath loud sound from nose

POSE FOR 20 BREATHS

Nadi Shodhana

MIND WHAT'S HAPPENING
Relaxed and Cool.

BODY WHERE IS THE EFFECT
Central Nervous System.

ATTENTION
On the third eye.

BREATH
Soft, silent breathing.

SEQUENCE

- Sit comfortably with spine erect.
- Keep the left hand in chin mudra. Use the right hand for switching the nostrils. Begin by breathing in and breathing out and bringing the awareness to the breath.
- Now gently touch the thumb to the right nostril, and breathe in softly from the left nostril. Anchor the index finger and middle finger on or near the third eye.
- Gently touch the ring finger to the left nostril and let go the thumb and release the breath from the right nostril.
- Now maintain the fingers position and breathe in from the right. Reverse the fingers and breathe out from the left.
- From left to right and back to left makes one round.
- Continue for 9 rounds or 5 minutes whichever is later.
- In the end, Breathe OUT from the LEFT and bring the hand down.

Adjust yourself, realign your muscles, then sit in silence for few seconds before opening the eyes.

COUNTER POSE = Smile Pose

7 Steps 7 Minutes

7 ASPECTS

Better to take out time for deep breathing every day.

- Better to learn breath control from a Master.
- Devote at least 7 minutes.

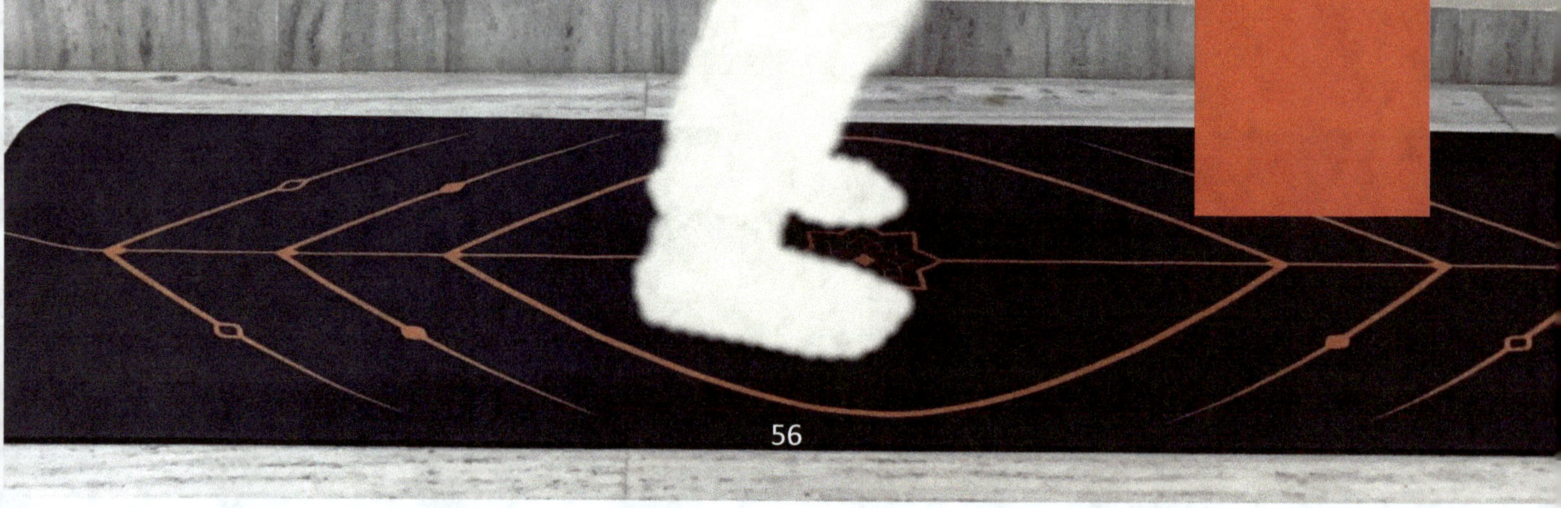

ALTERNATE

NOSTRIL

NADI SHODANA

BREATH IS KEY

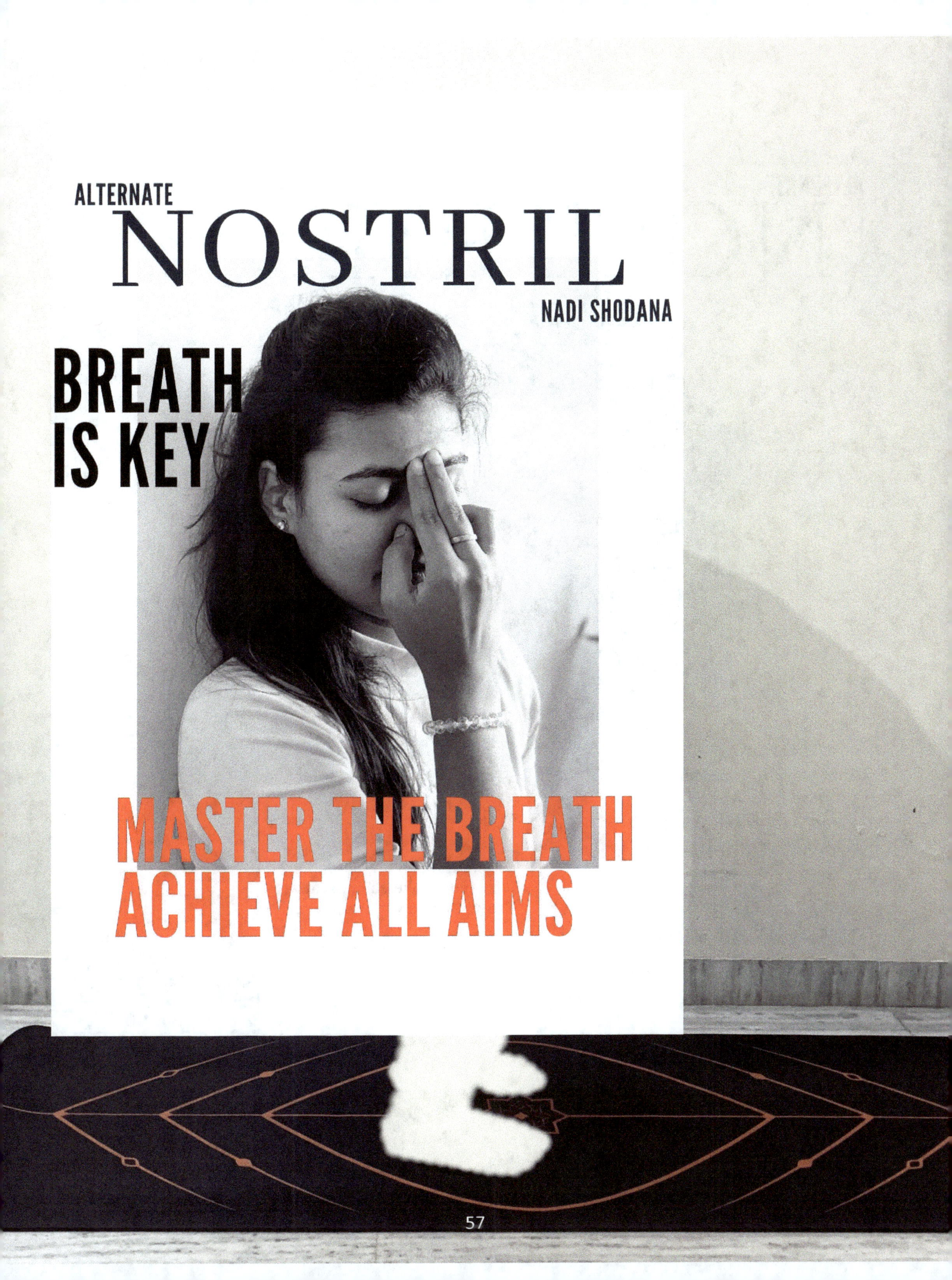

MASTER THE BREATH ACHIEVE ALL AIMS

ALTERNATE

NOSTRIL

NADI SHODANA

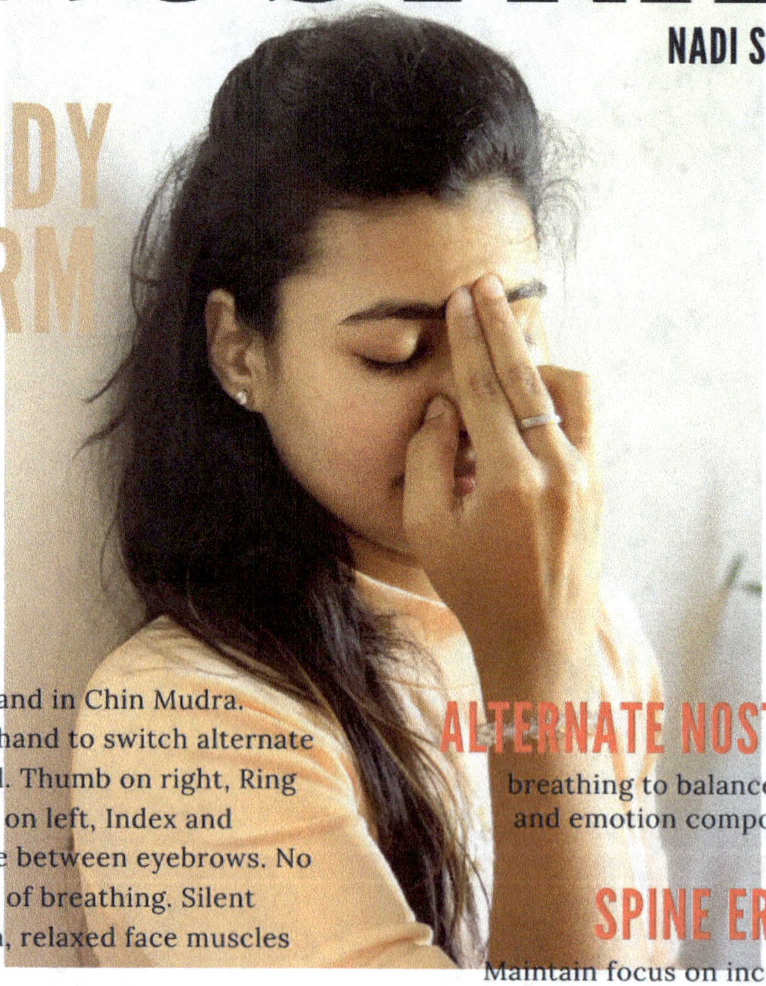

BODY FIRM

Left hand in Chin Mudra. Right hand to switch alternate nostril. Thumb on right, Ring finger on left, Index and Middle between eyebrows. No sound of breathing. Silent breath, relaxed face muscles

ALTERNATE NOSTRIL

breathing to balance logic and emotion components

SPINE ERECT

Maintain focus on incoming outgoing, make each breath smooth s l o w quiver-free

POSE FOR 9 ROUNDS OF BREATH

Pratyahara Inward Turn

PATANJALI YOGA SUTRAS

स्व–विषया–सम्प्रयोगे चित्तस्य स्वरूप–अनुकार इवेन्द्रियाणां प्रत्याहारः ॥ २.५४॥

svaviṣayāsamprayoge cittasya svarūpānukāra ivendriyāṇāṁ pratyāhāraḥ ॥

2.54 Pratyahara is like making the Senses follow_the essential_nature_of_the_mind by separating them from their corresponding objects

pratyāhāra = *Alternate Food for the Senses = for turning the Senses Inwards = mechanism of Withdrawing the senses*

Just like a tortoise withdraws its limbs inside, so in Pratyahara we withdraw the senses inwards, by giving the senses an alternative.

Pratyahara is a mechanism of controlling the outward movement of sense organs like sight, sound, etc. by giving them something inside the body to dwell upon, likewise by dancing and singing, or engaging in any creative fine arts process.

Dharana Concentration

PATANJALI YOGA SUTRAS

देश–बन्धश्चित्तस्य धारणा ॥ ३.१ ॥ deśabandhaścittasya dhāraṇā ॥

3.1 Dharana is Fixing the mind at a place

dhāraṇā = *Concentration is holding the mind at a particular place.*
e.g. Bringing the focus to the third-eye is Dharana.
e.g. Concentration on baking the cake is Dharana.

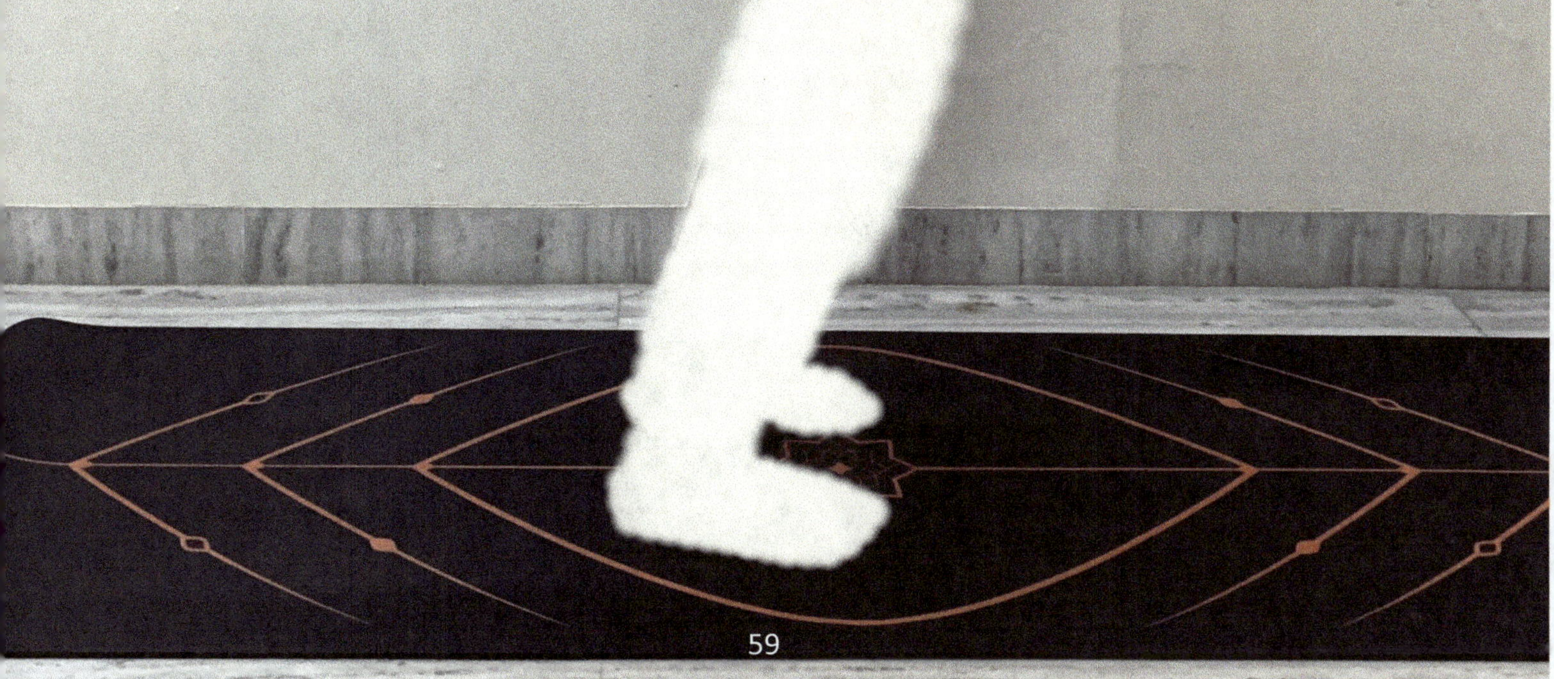

2 Meditation Dhyana

PATANJALI YOGA SUTRAS

तत्र प्रत्ययैकतानता ध्यानम् ॥ ३.२॥ tatra pratyayaikatānatā dhyānam ॥

3.2 There the unbroken flow of similar thoughts is Dhyana

dhyāna = *Contemplation. Is having a stream of like thoughts towards some topic, object, matter or subject, without consciously trying. Bringing the mind to the present moment.*
e.g. Having prolonged thoughts regarding third-eye, Ajna Chakra, between the eye-brows, etc. is Dhyana.
e.g. Repeatedly having thoughts regarding what to bake for the birthday party is Dhyana.

After a while, when one is not holding the mind, yet it stays, it is called Dhyana or Contemplation.

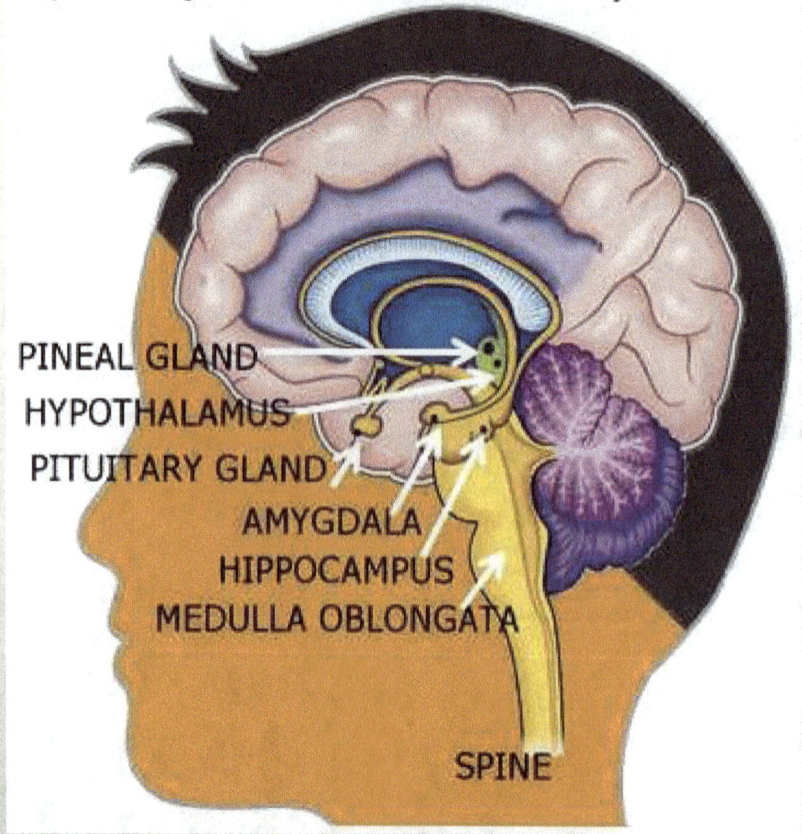

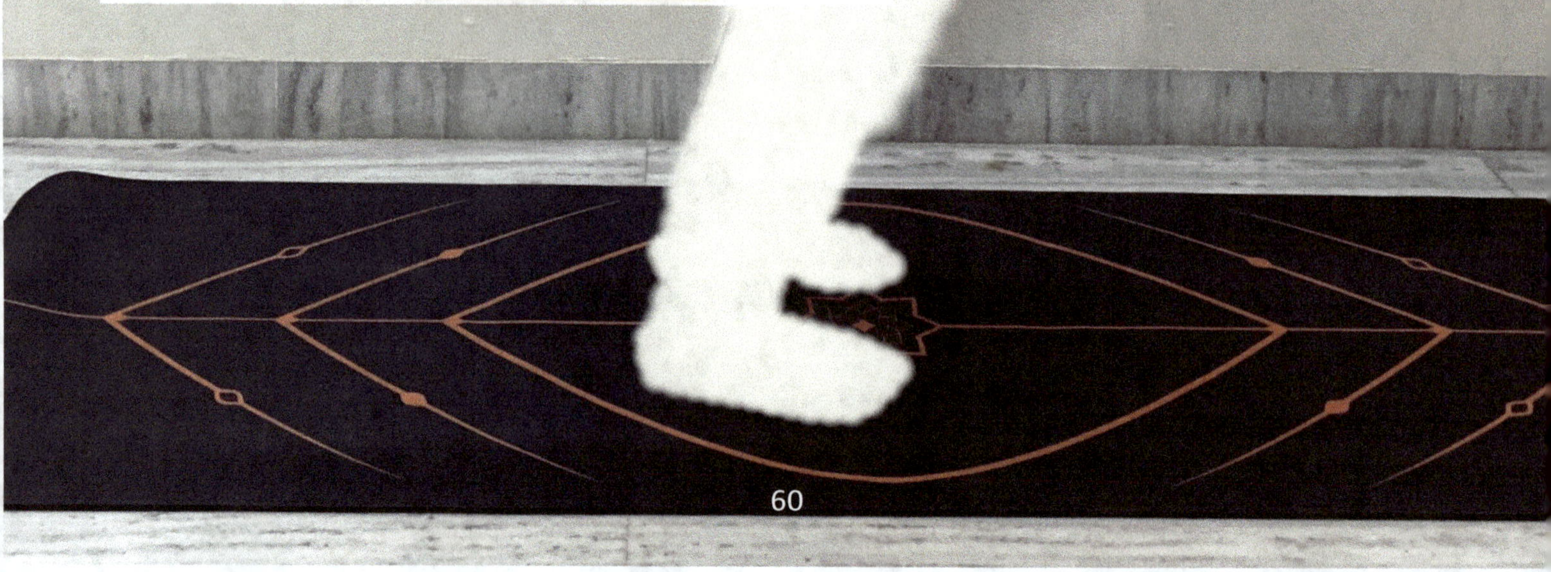

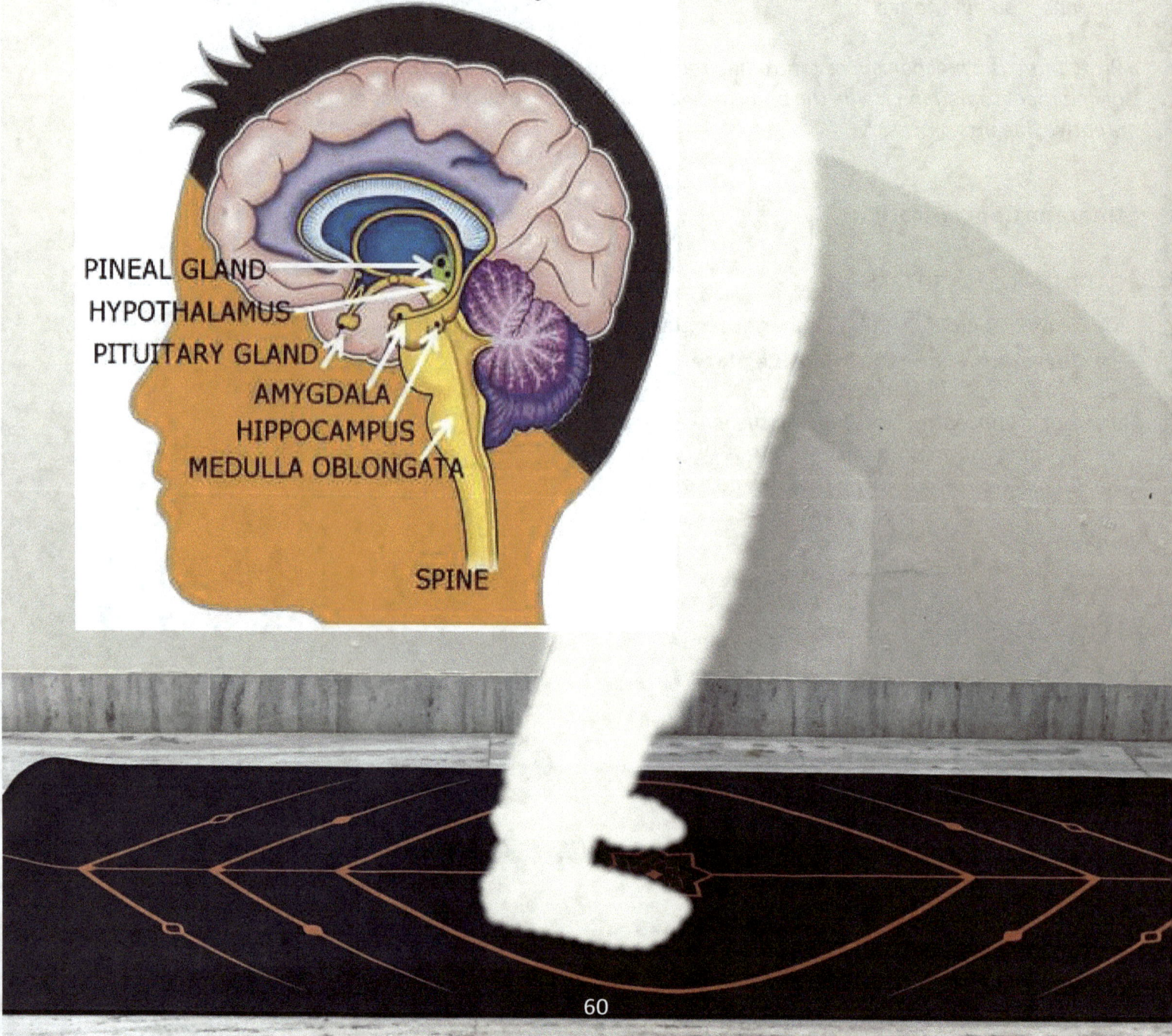

Importance of Guided Meditation

For being able to Meditate, we need an accomplished teacher. Only from the one who has attained the state of deep Samadhi, can one be initiated into Meditation. Gurudev Sri Sri Ravi Shankar has effortlessly guided millions to achieve that pristine state of absolute stillness in the mind. To hear him guide one is to truly experience that rare bliss that otherwise proves elusive even to advanced practitioners. Important areas in the Brain and words used by Gurudev during Meditation. **Hypothalamus** is the very center of the brain, often referred to as the Brahmarandra in the Vedic literature. Similarly **Amygdala** is the chief controller of subtle energy channels, while the **pineal** is the chief controller of physical body. **Pituitary** is the master of the endocrine system.
https://isha.sadhguru.org/in/en/wisdom/article/brahmarandhra-passage-for-life

Hari Om Meditation

A deep effortless chakra cleansing meditation by chanting HARI OM at each of the seven chakras.
HINDI https://www.youtube.com/watch?v=qKt9jWvzd60
ENGLISH https://www.youtube.com/watch?v=Mrk_V68V6UE

Pancakosha Meditation

Honoring the five sheaths and transcending them to attain pure bliss.
ENGLISH https://www.youtube.com/watch?v=25pGz8MEmEQ
HINDI https://www.youtube.com/watch?v=yJzkB5uFxXg

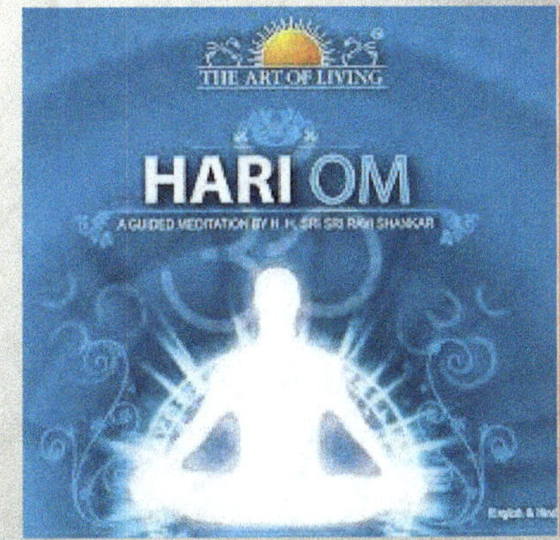

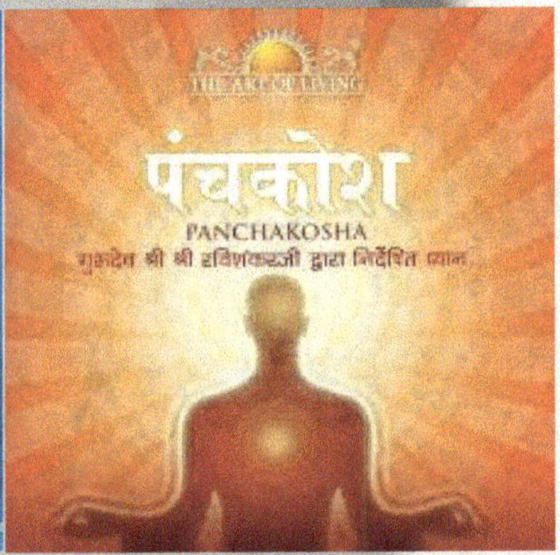

Gurudev has repeatedly emphasized on Meditation as the principal Yogic practice. It is enjoined to be done twice a day for 10 to 20 minutes to harmonize the entire BODY MIND complex. It certainly helps attain the supreme state of nirvana. It is also highly recommended to enable anyone to perform to peak capacity on the materialistic front and keep all illnesses at bay.
https://www.srisriravishankar.org/live/

The Sahaj Samadhi Meditation from the Art of Living is a simple technique to discover one's talents and express oneself beautifully in the world. https://www.artofliving.org/in-en/art-of-meditation-program

महामुद्रा महाबन्धो महावेधश्च खेचरी।

उड्डीयानं मूलबन्धश्च बन्धो जालन्धराभिधः ॥ ३.६॥ Hatha Yoga Pradipika

mahāmudrā mahābandho mahāvedhaśca khecarī ।

uḍḍīyānaṃ mūlabandhaśca bandho jālandharābhidhaḥ ॥ 3.6 ॥

3.6

The practice of Mudras and Bandhas has a great effect on the subtle channels within the body, destroying the knots and awakening the kundalini shakti.

Uddiyan Bandha, Moolabandha, and Jalandhar bandha are named here, and held together these three comprise the maha bandha or great lock.

Samadhi Transcendental State

PATANJALI YOGA SUTRAS

तदेव अर्थ–मात्र–निर्भासं स्वरूप–शून्यम् इव समाधिः ॥ ३.३॥

tadevārthamātranirbhāsaṁ svarūpaśūnyamiva samādhiḥ ॥

3.3 Samadhi is illumination of that meaning only, having lost all notion

samādhi = *Deep Meditation occurs when the focus has dissolved, thoughts have vanished, personality has evaporated, and only an awareness lingers.*

Samadhi *is when the notion of body and mind vanishes and only a faint yet alert awareness remains.*

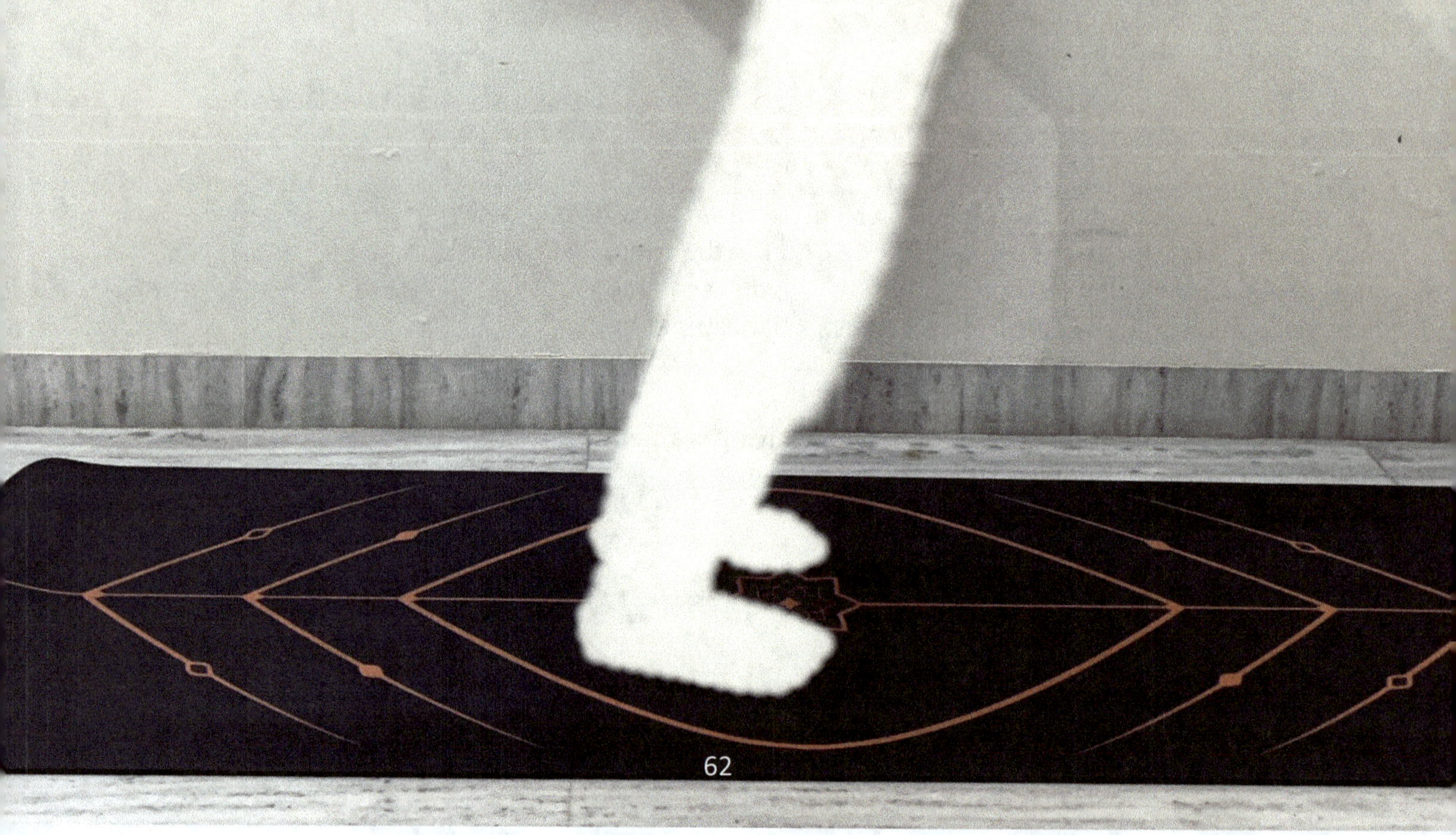

3 Walking

A brisk walk in fresh air for 40 minutes is a complete YOGA practice in itself, provided one is not carrying bags, phones, and accessories that cause strain on one set of muscles and make the posture uneven or the mind distracted.

Gossiping with friends during a walk might reduce its value, however if that helps in regularity, then let it be.

7 Steps 7 Minutes

7 ASPECTS

Walking is a wholesome Art.

- It is the one practice that should not be shelved.
- Walk for at least 7 minutes.

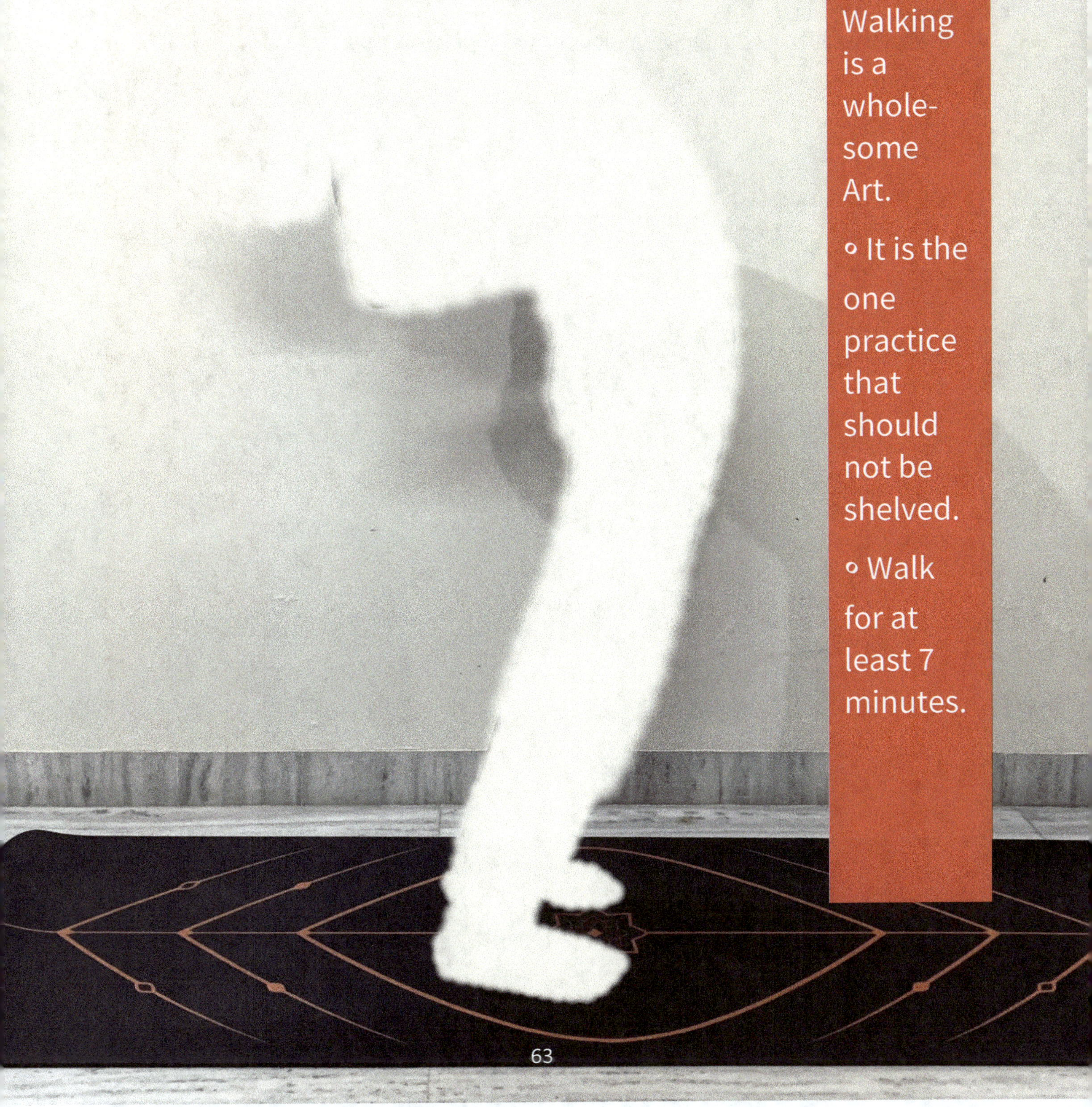

5 Outdoor Sports

Cycling, Jogging, Swimming, and playing Badminton, Football, Lawn Tennis, Cricket are excellent ways to be fit, cheerful, and successful.

Developing team spirit and social acceptance and improving confidence and personality are natural byproducts of outdoor sports.

https://www.olympic.org/
https://www.verywellfamily.com/great-outdoor-games-for-kids-620396

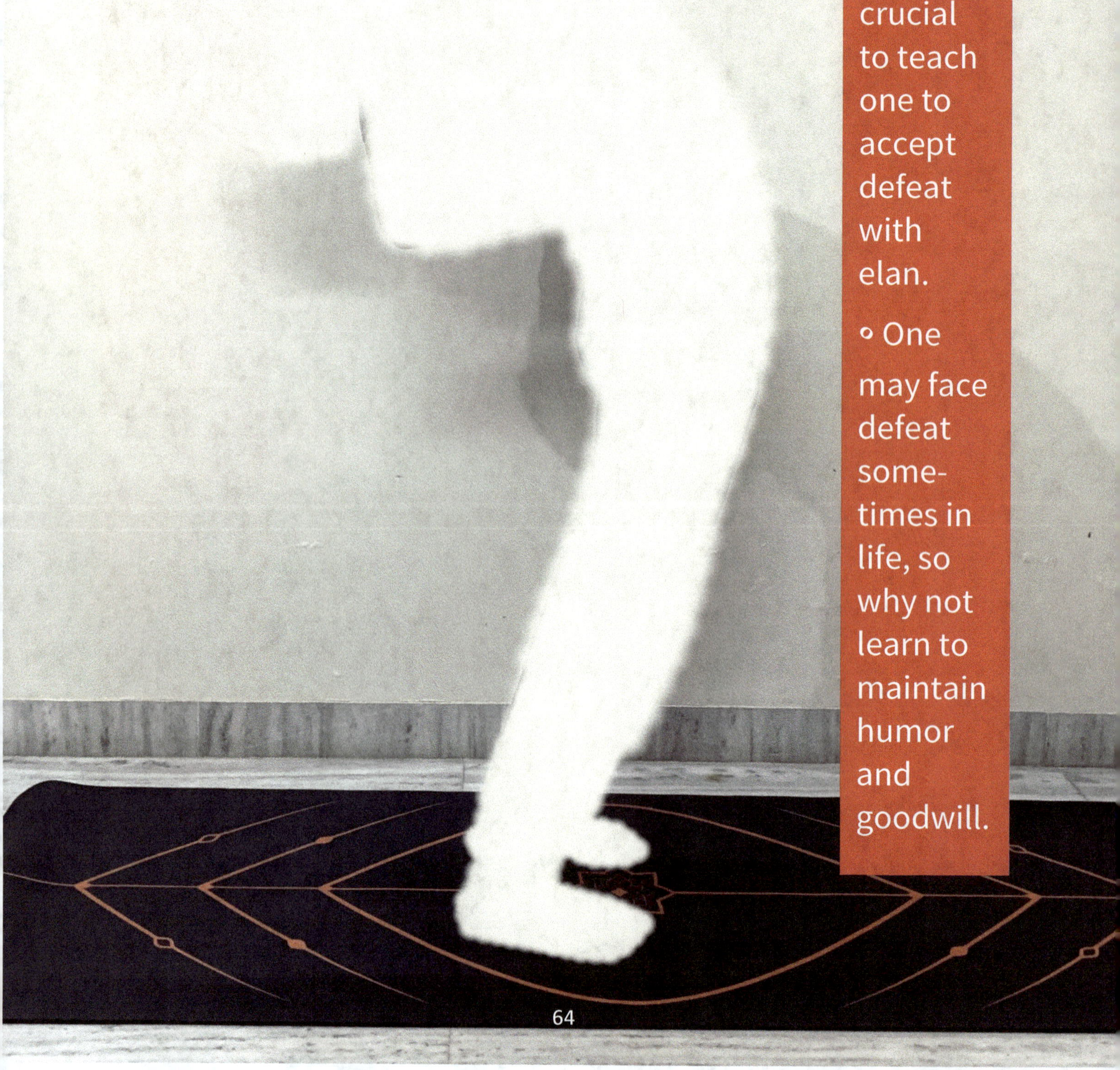

7 Steps 7 Minutes

7 ASPECTS

Sports is crucial to teach one to accept defeat with elan.

- One may face defeat sometimes in life, so why not learn to maintain humor and goodwill.

6 Havan

Puja Havan Satsang Aarti.

Coming together and praying can take many forms. Festivals and Celebrations that occur every month should be fully partaken of and enjoyed. It is both the fruit and the reward of our human existence.

Guru Puja is such a graceful offering that takes 7 minutes.

https://www.artofliving.org/in-en/guru-puja-1
https://www.youtube.com/watch?v=vO1Cc8F99Vo

https://vaidicpujas.org/
http://homatherapy.org/

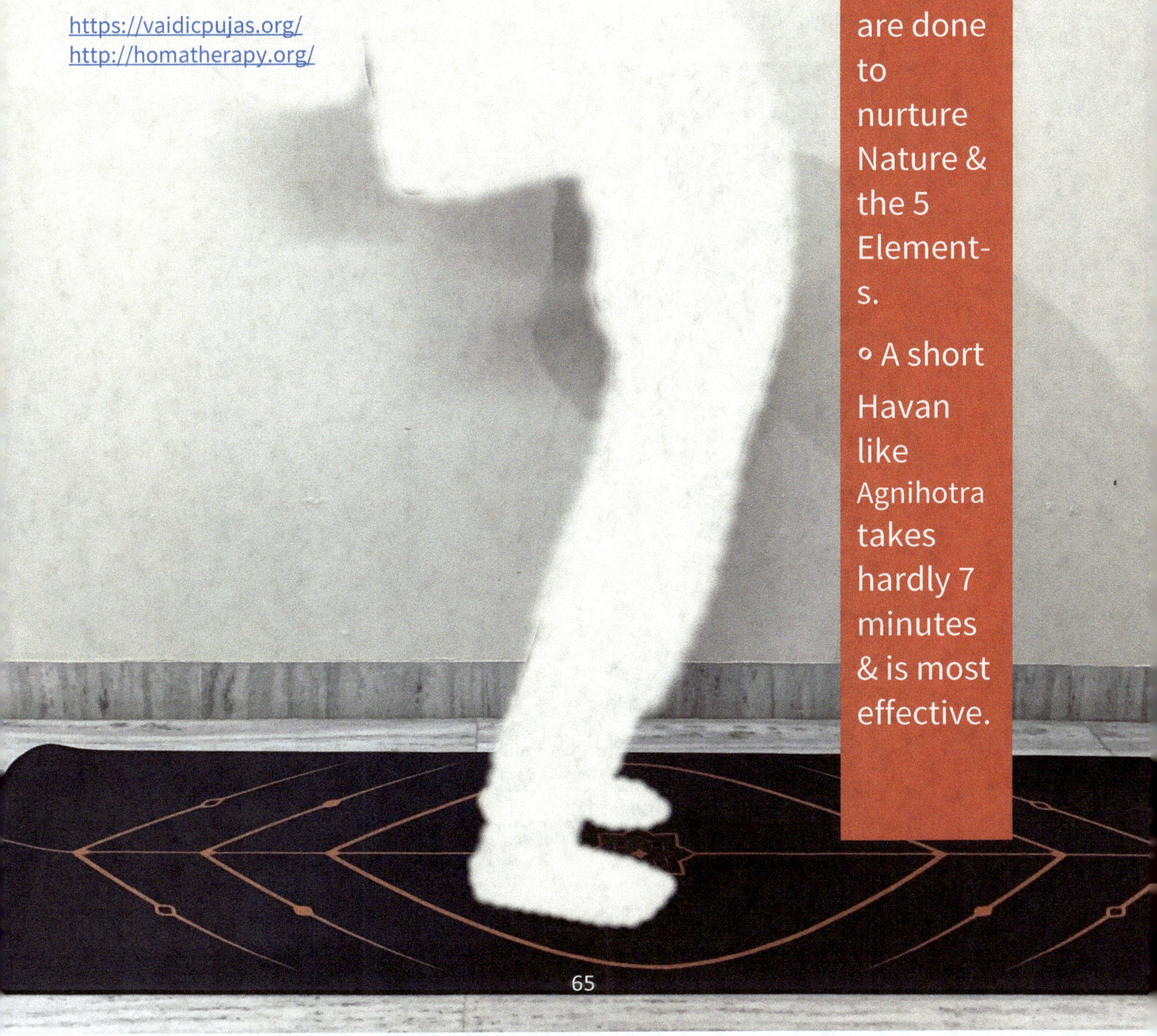

7 Steps 7 Minutes

7 ASPECTS

HAVAN

- Yagyas are done to nurture Nature & the 5 Elements.
- A short Havan like Agnihotra takes hardly 7 minutes & is most effective.

Regular Habits

Watch your Tongue

Refrain from using harsh, cruel, cutting or bitter words. Keep a strict watch on the tongue. It is an integral part of Yogic Lifestyle.

Prayer Chanting and Singing

Chanting aloud mantras and verses and singing hymns keeps the brain youthful, the senses alert and memory sharp.

Om Namah Shivaya
https://www.youtube.com/watch?v=CWWwvF556w8

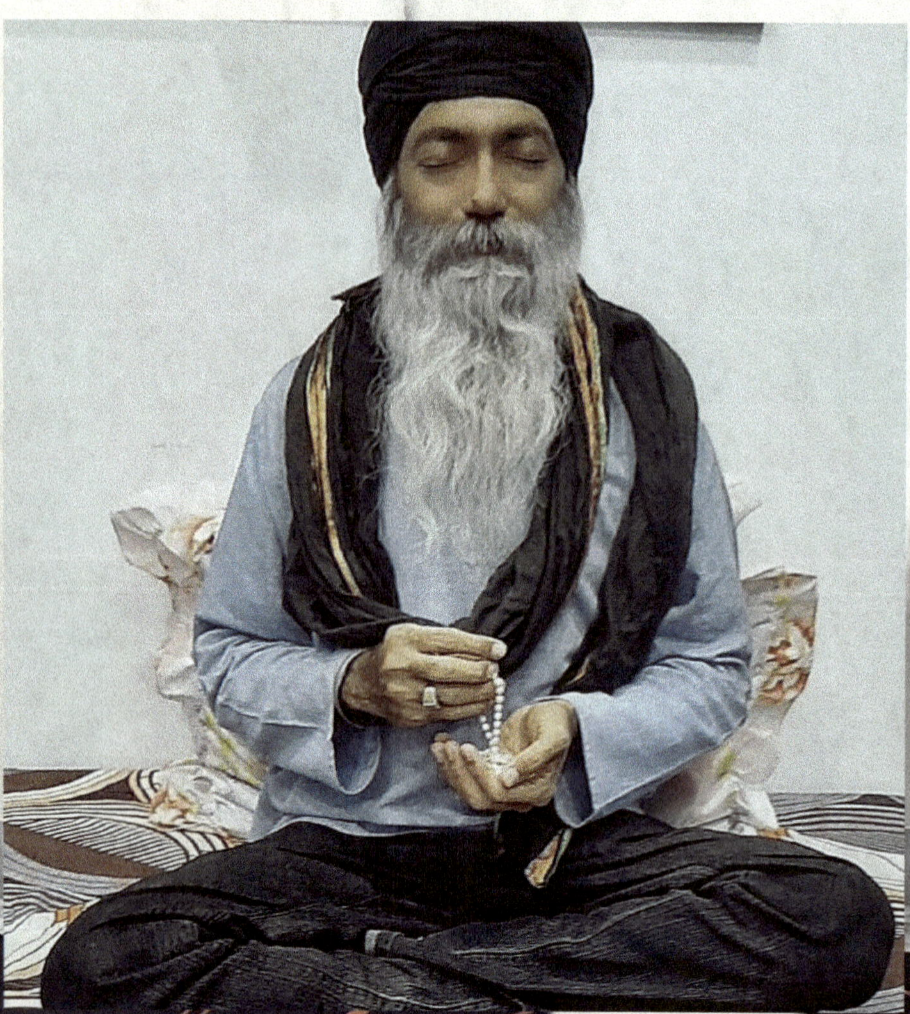

Not to be missed is Prayer. Start at a young age and reap its incredible effects, especially in pressing moments.

Diet

Yoga practice has its two right hand men – Diet and Ayurveda.
Sattvic freshly cooked. According to ayurvedic constitution. Lots of salads, soups, juices. Less of salt and sugar. Use desi cow ghee or mustard oil or virgin coconut oil or ground oil for cooking. Avoid white sugar, refined oils, A1 milk products, packaged foods, esoteric non-seasonal items. Go for A2 milk. Local Seasonal fruits and veggies. Making an effort to find out and use chemical free food products.
http://www.djjs.org/kamdhenu/initiatives

Marma, Meru Chikitsa, Craniosacral Therapy Reflexology

These wonderful therapies have recently caught the attention of the general public as safe, non-invasive, suitable for all healing methodologies.

https://www.artofliving.org/in-en/wellness/sri-sri-marma
https://www.srisritattvapanchakarma.com/product/meru-chikitsa/
https://www.youtube.com/watch?v=nVDBbOChuB0
https://www.artofliving.org/in-en/lifestyle/well-being/everything-you-wanted-to-know-about-craniosacral-therapy

Panchakarma

These traditional detox therapies make the body feel very fresh, rejuvenated, cleansed and alive. All of us must attend panchakarma sessions at least couple of times a year. They are safe and can give miraculous healing. Many stubborn illnesses can be effectively managed and health can be brought back on track by Panchakarma.
https://www.artofliving.org/in-en/ayurveda/sri-sri-ayurveda-panchakarma
https://www.srisritattvapanchakarma.com/

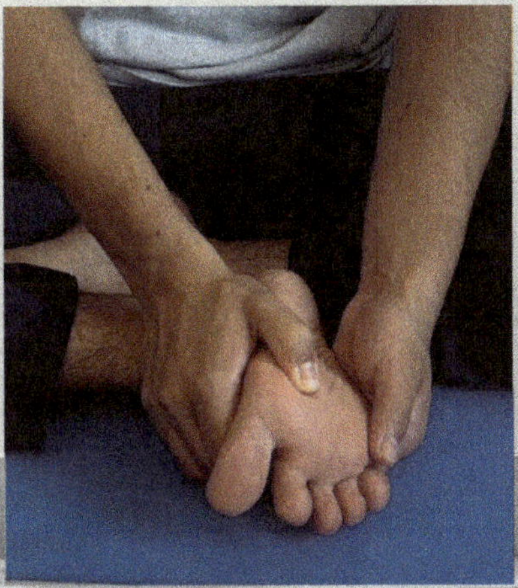

Pressing points on the feet

https://www.youtube.com/watch?v=yqx4YIr6PQs

https://en.wikipedia.org/wiki/Reflexology

Eye care & Tooth care

Liquid Eyes and Shining Teeth are what make us appear more beautiful. These help maintain our confidence and acceptance in society.

Good eyesight and healthy teeth and gums are visible to all around us, making them potent winners during interviews and match-making. That in turn results in higher efficiency and greater success in life.

It helps to wash eyes with Triphala water regularly. Doing 20 minutes of eye exercises in sunlight is highly recommended, especially at dawn or dusk when the sunrays are cool.

https://www.srisritattvapanchakarma.com/eye-care/
https://www.artofliving.org/in-en/ayurveda/therapies/keep-your-eye-healthy-and-strong-part-1

With the rapid changes in food and eating habits, no longer is toothpaste good enough. We must add toothpowder, dantmanjan and datun, and also concoctions like alum water in our daily tooth-brushing regimen. These go a long way in preventing mouth illnesses and help maintain healthy teeth and strong gums.

It also makes sense to inculcate the habit of brushing twice a day.
https://www.mayoclinic.org/healthy-lifestyle/adult-health/in-depth/dental/art-20045536

Patanjali Yoga Sutras

तपःस्वाध्यायेश्वरप्रणिधानानि क्रियायोगः ॥ २.१ ॥

tapaḥsvādhyāyeśvarapraṇidhānāni kriyāyogaḥ ॥ 2.1 ॥

तपः–स्वाध्याय–ईश्वरप्रणिधानानि क्रिया–योगः ।

Tapas, Svādhyāya and Ishvarpranidhana are directives for Yoga

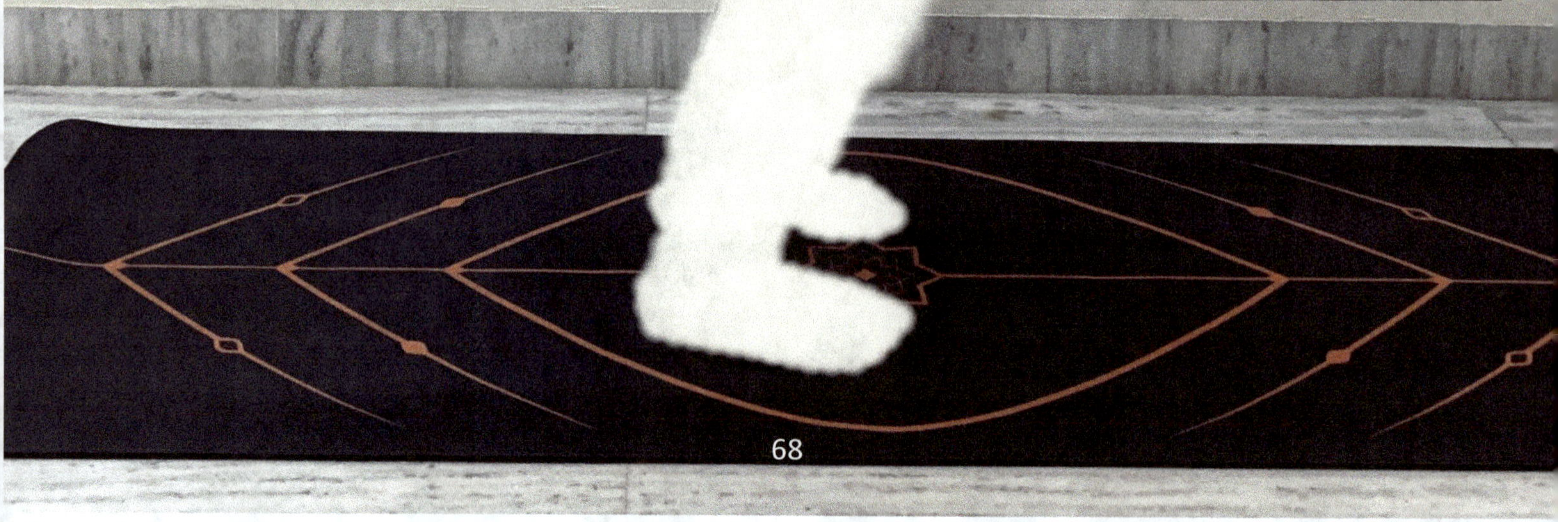

Mudra and Bandha

Mahā Mudra

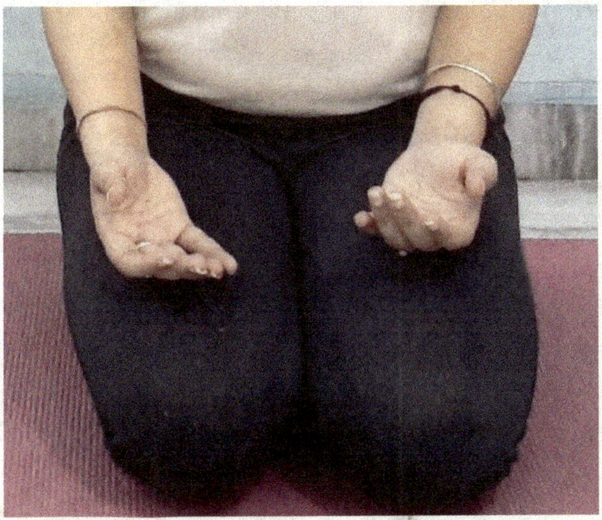

Various hand gestures are employed to make or break the subtle nadi circuits in the body, and direct prana effectively to cure and strengthen internal organs.

Open palms simply and loosely kept on the knees or in the lap, open towards the sky, to harness and soak in the cosmic energies.

Mahā Bandha

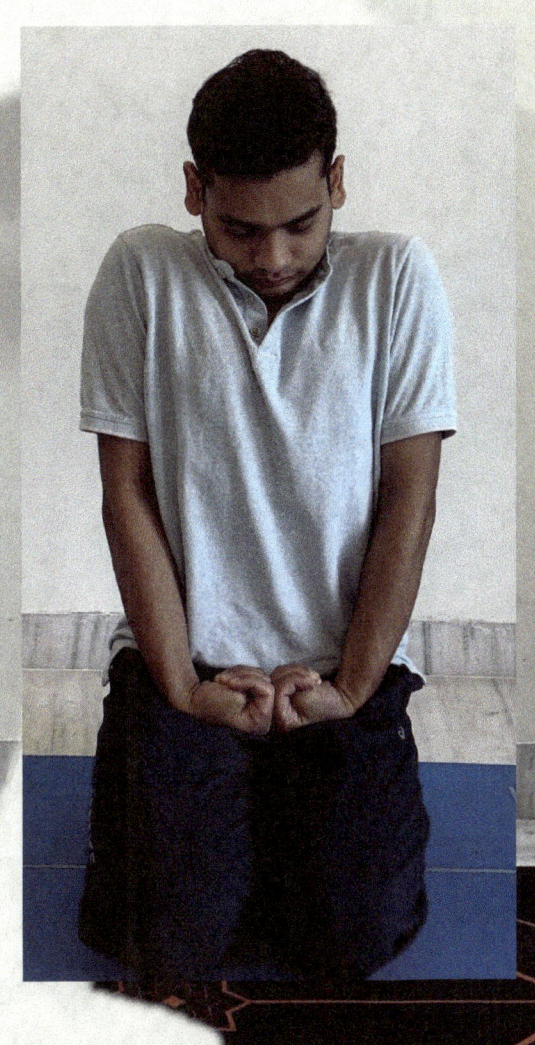

Breathe in, then
Sequential application of **Moola**, **Uddiyan**, and **Jalandhar** Bandhas respectively.

Palms in Adi Mudra, with Knuckles touching, nails facing upward.

Elbows straight, shoulders upped.

Breath retained inside for few seconds comfortably.

Slowly release the Jalandhar bandha, then while exhaling release Uddiyan and finally the Moolabandha.

Yoga is a Family thing

Yoga is not bound to girls or boys, teenagers or adults. Yoga is for grandparents and children both.

All members of a family can practice Yoga regularly, making their individual mix-and-match of asana and pranayama. And they can practice Meditation and Prayer and Singing as a group.

Yoga is not limited to the Orient, it is equally enjoyed in the Occident

Babies and young children of all races and cultures and ethnic backgrounds do most of the asanas while growing up.

Open your eyes and notice this entrancing fact. They even do many mudras. And the result??? We all see the exuberance, agility, smiling countenance of young children and wonder where their energy and godliness comes from? It is their inherent tendency to perform asanas, mudras, and breathing patterns that are direct Yogic practices.

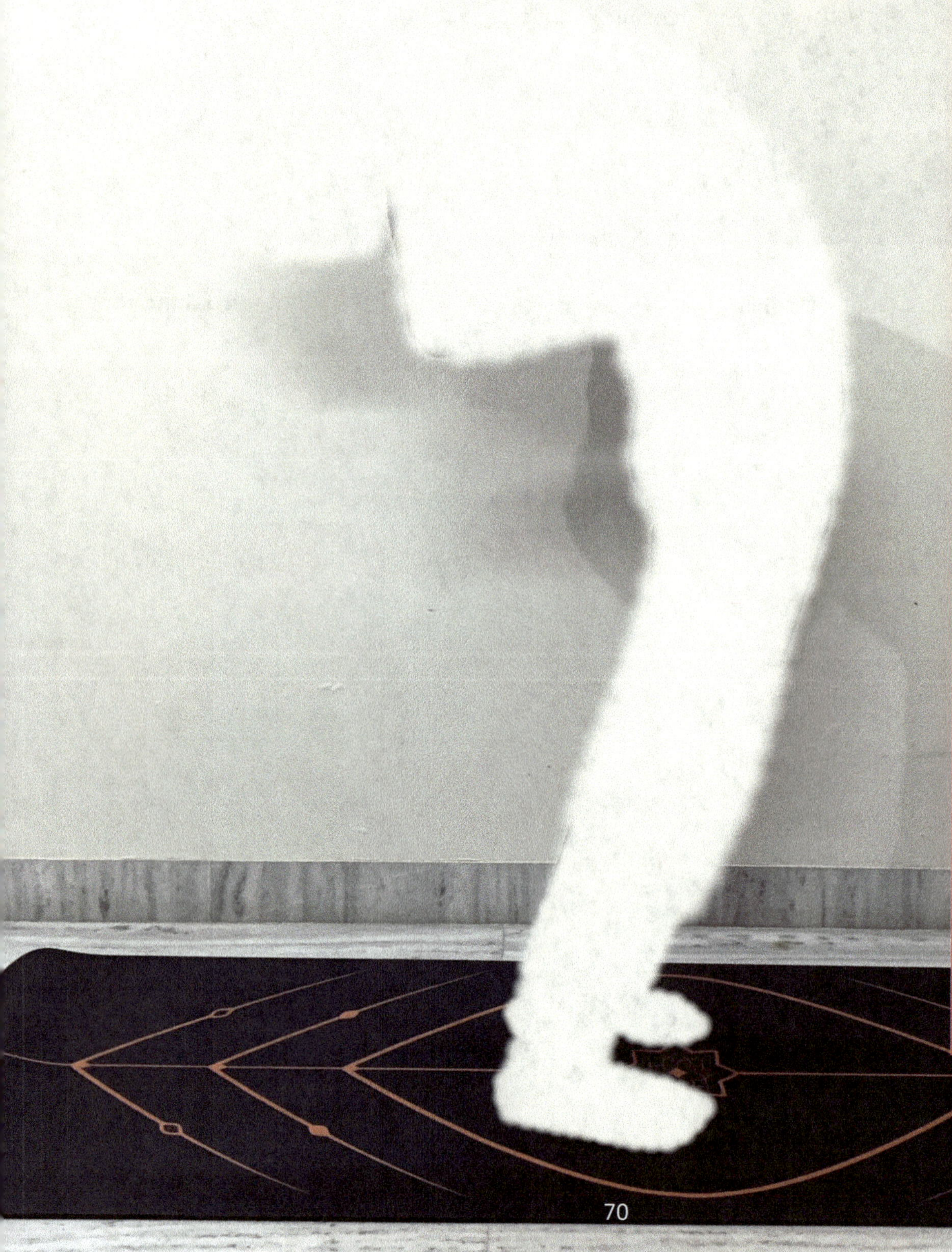

7 Steps 7 Minutes

7 ASPECTS

TONGUE

- Watch your tongue!
- Modulate your speech.
- Be soft spoken.
- A kind tongue is YOGA at its best.

Asana Handout

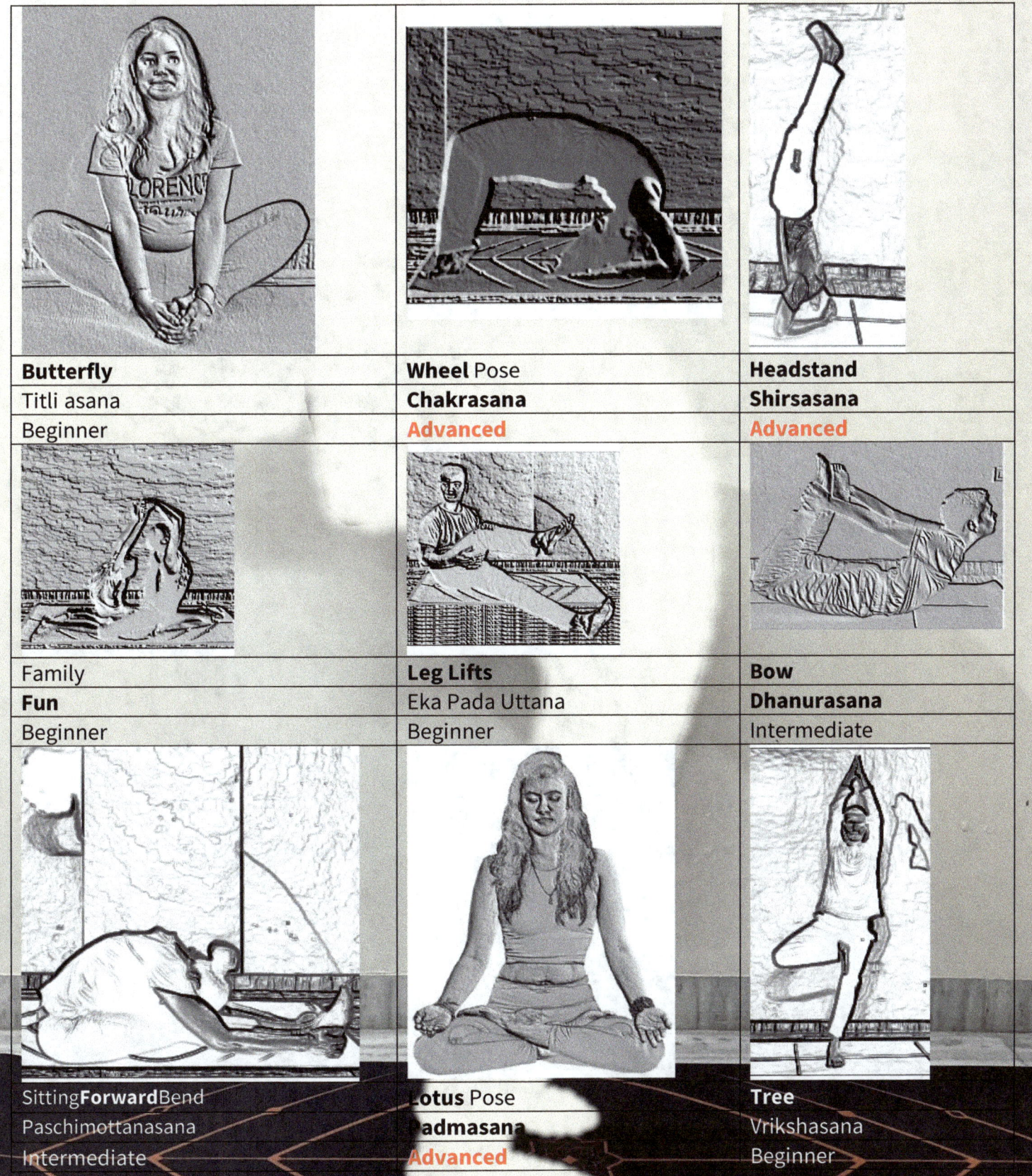

		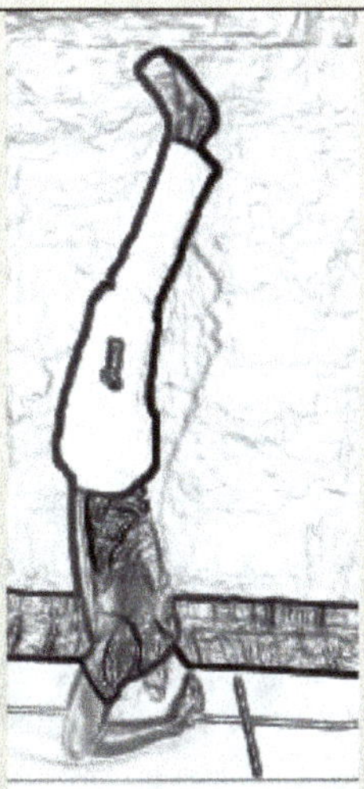
Butterfly	**Wheel** Pose	**Headstand**
Titli asana	**Chakrasana**	**Shirsasana**
Beginner	**Advanced**	**Advanced**
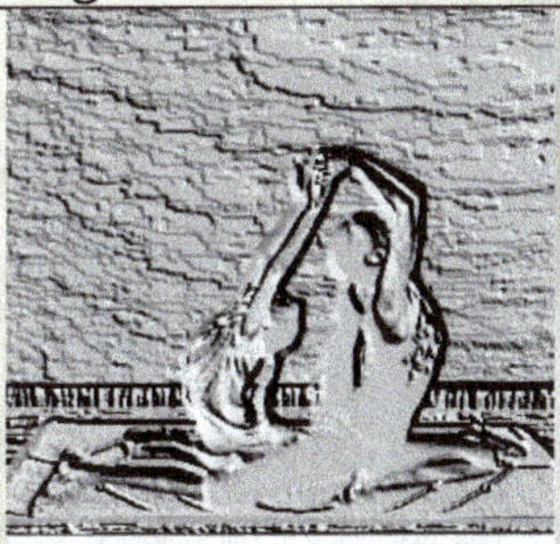	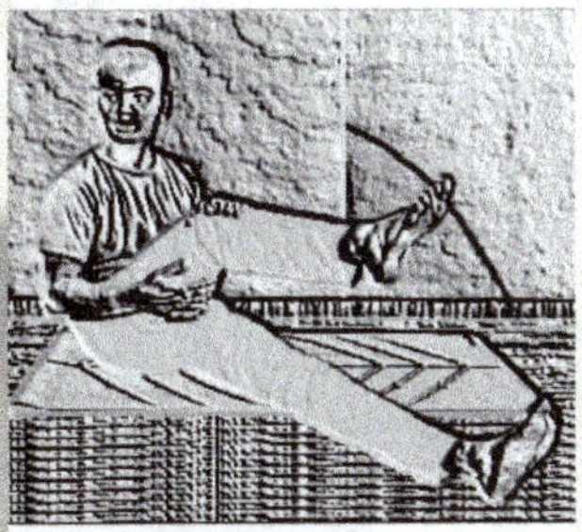	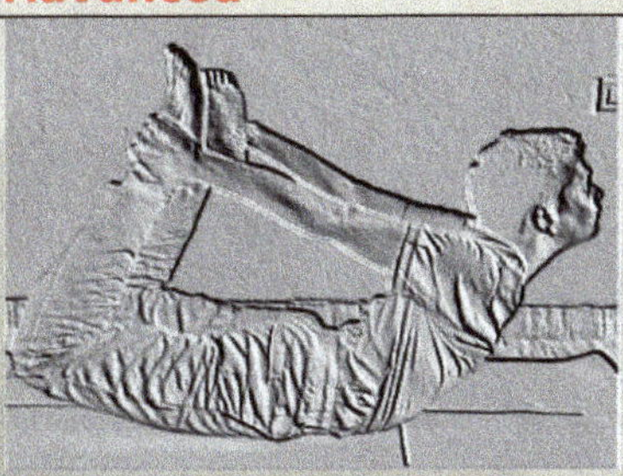
Family	**Leg Lifts**	**Bow**
Fun	Eka Pada Uttana	**Dhanurasana**
Beginner	Beginner	Intermediate
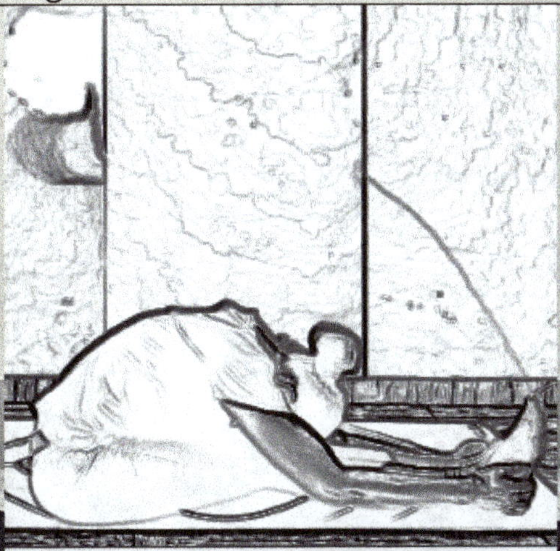		
Sitting**Forward**Bend	**Lotus** Pose	**Tree**
Paschimottanasana	**Padmasana**	Vrikshasana
Intermediate	**Advanced**	Beginner

Wall Support

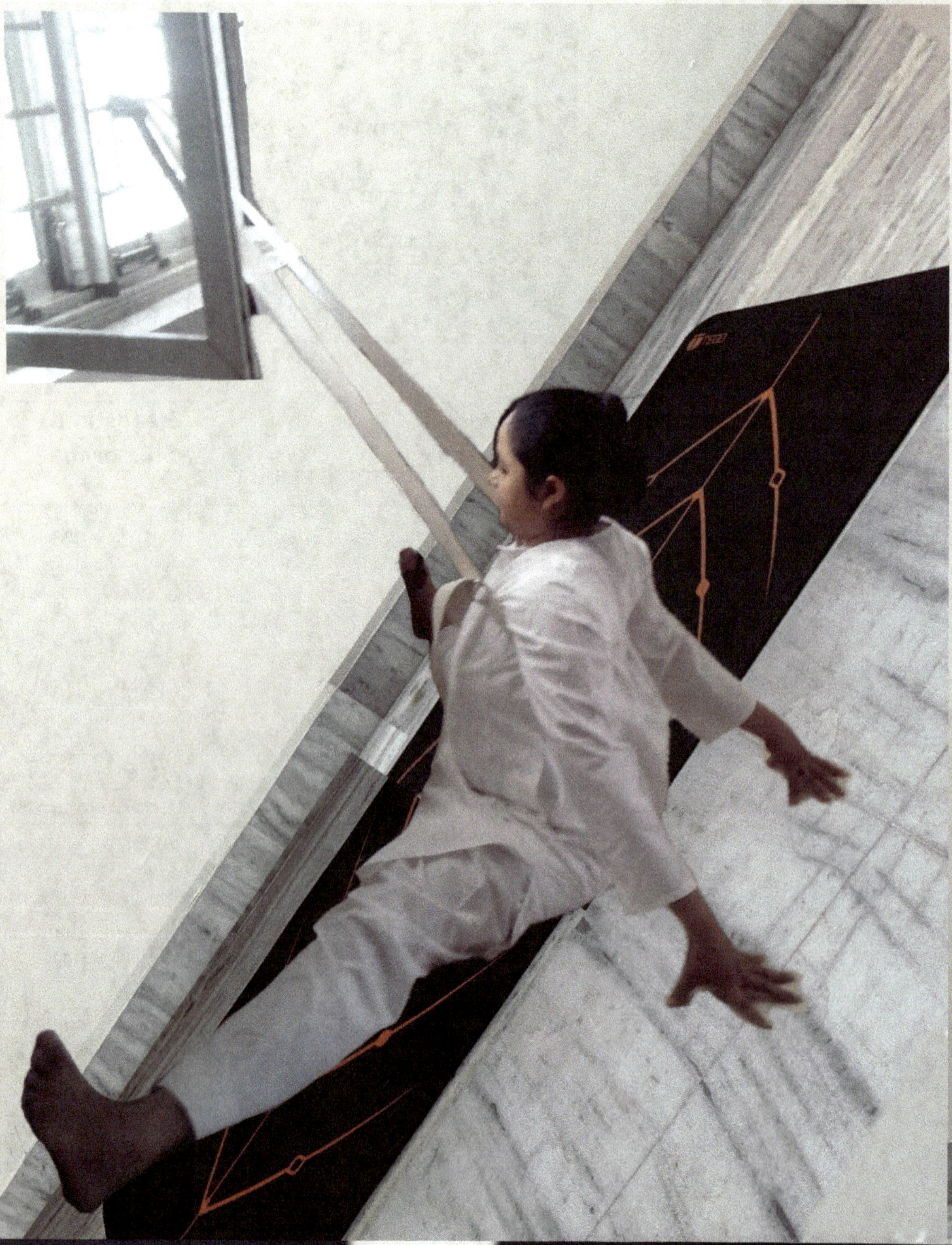

Using Wall Support can prevent injury and significantly increase confidence in the practice.

Traditional Texts

Yoga Vasistha

https://www.shivabalayogi.org/Books/Yoga_Vasistha.htm
http://swamivenkatesananda.org/books?id=4
https://archive.org/details/TheYogaVasisthaOfValmikiINirnayaSagarPress

यतः सर्वाणि भूतानि प्रतिभान्ति स्थितानि च ।

यत्रैवोपशमं यान्ति तस्मै सत्यात्मने नमः ॥ १॥

ज्ञाता ज्ञानं तथा ज्ञेयं द्रष्टा दर्शनदृश्यभूः ।

कर्ता हेतुः क्रिया यस्मात् तस्मै ज्ञप्त्यात्मने नमः ॥ २॥

स्फुरन्ति सीकरा यस्माद् आनन्दस्याम्बरेऽवनौ ।

सर्वेषां जीवनं तस्मै ब्रह्मानन्दात्मने नमः ॥ ३॥

yataḥ sarvāṇi bhūtāni pratibhānti sthitāni ca |

yatraivopaśamaṃ yānti tasmai satyātmane namaḥ || 1||

jñātā jñānaṃ tathā jñeyaṃ draṣṭā darśanadṛśyabhūḥ |

kartā hetuḥ kriyā yasmāt tasmai jñaptyātmane namaḥ || 2||

sphuranti sīkarā yasmād ānandasyāmbare'vanau |

sarveṣāṃ jīvanaṃ tasmai brahmānandātmane namaḥ || 3||

1. To that inviolable Truth in whom is cradled the cosmos,
   is offered my sincere salutation.

2. To that all knowing Self in whom the transactional plays are enacted, is offered my deepest gratitude.

3. To that all fulfilling pleasure giving splendorous Divinity,
   is offered my soul's delight.

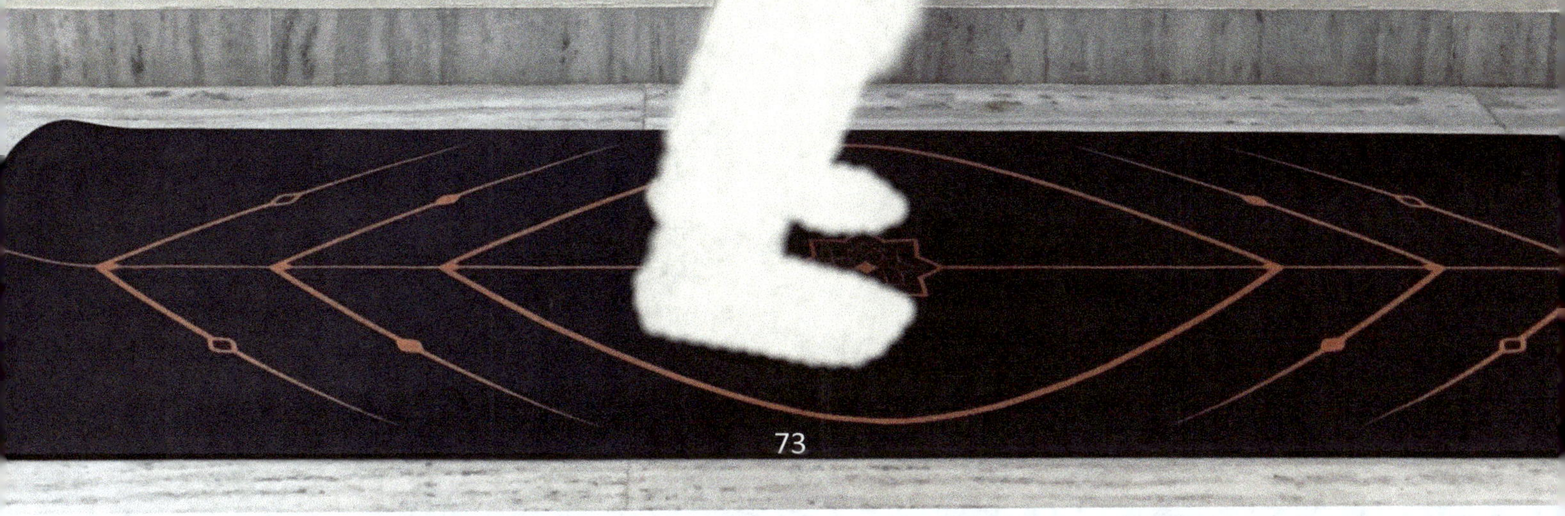

Bhagavad Gita

https://www.amazon.in/dp/B0732Z17TF
https://www.amazon.in/dp/B07JF9W71F/
https://live.artofliving.org/bhagavad-gita

मत्तः परतरं नान्यत् , किञ्चिद् अस्ति धनञ्जय ।

मयि सर्वमिदं प्रोतम् , सूत्रे मणिगणा इव ॥ ७.७

mattaḥ parataraṁ nānyat , kiñcid asti dhanañjaya ।

mayi sarvamidaṁ protam , sūtre maṇigaṇā iva ॥ 7.7

7.7
The highest Truth supports all and
is present in all and everything.

You may loosely think of the Truth
as a chain on which pearls are strung
to form a necklace.

बुद्धियुक्तो जहातीह , उभे सुकृतदुष्कृते ।

तस्माद् योगाय युज्यस्व , योगः कर्मसु कौशलम् ॥ २.५०

buddhiyukto jahātīha , ubhe sukṛtaduṣkṛte ।

tasmād yogāya yujyasva , yogaḥ karmasu kauśalam ॥ 2.50

2.50
The one who gives his 100%
gets rid of all bias and temptation.

Therefore put your heart and soul
in your deeds.

Skill in Action is called Yoga.
Dexterity is another name for yogic living.

Patanjali Yoga Sutras

https://www.amazon.in/dp/B07331N54C
https://www.amazon.in/dp/B01M6WP0DZ
https://live.artofliving.org/patanjali-yoga-sutras

योगश्–चित्त-वृत्ति-निरोधः । १.२

Yogaś citta vṛtti nirodhaḥ । 1.2

1.2
Yogic Life entails a
Calming of the Processes
in the Mind

अभ्यासवैराग्याभ्यां तन्निरोधः । abhyāsavairāgyābhyāṁ tannirodhaḥ । 1.12

1.12
By the twin practices of
Abhyaasa and Vairagya –
Regular Practices and Dropping Entanglements
those are Tempered

तत्र स्थितौ यत्नोऽभ्यासः । tatra sthitau yatno'bhyāsaḥ । 1.13

1.13 Abhyaasa means being Steadfast in one's Effort

स तु दीर्घ–काल–नैरन्तर्य–सत्कारासेवितो दृढभूमिः ।

sa tu dīrghakālanairantaryasatkārāsevito dṛḍhabhūmiḥ । 1 14

1.14 And that when continuous over a long period of time with sincere devotion, establishes firm foundation

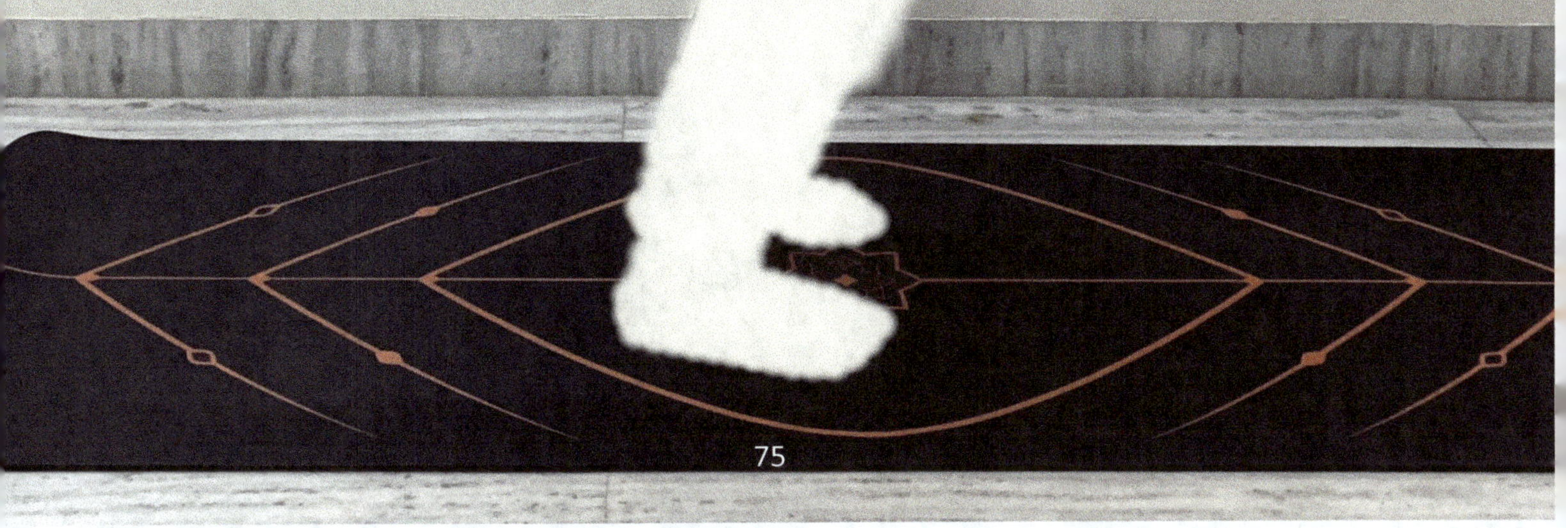

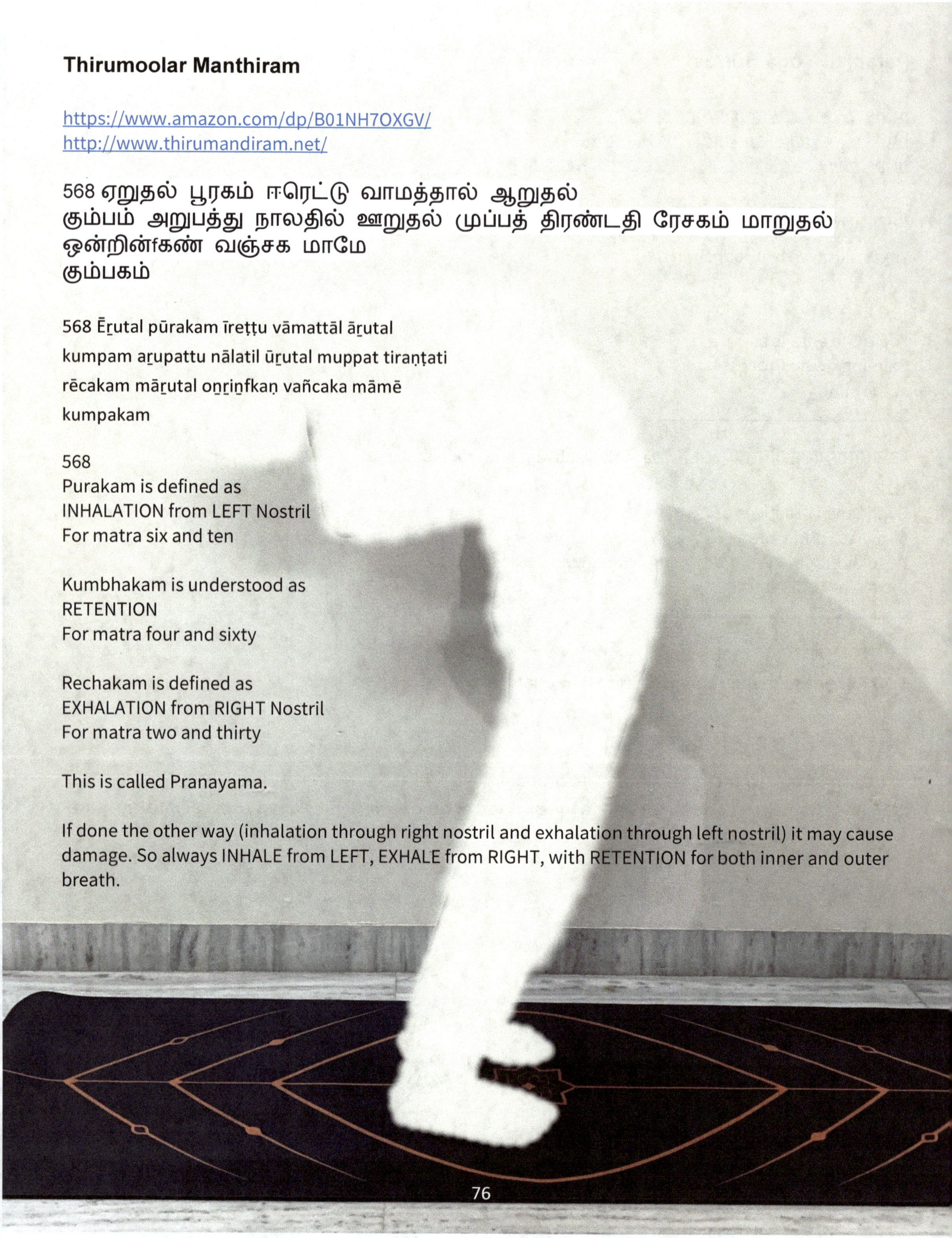

Thirumoolar Manthiram

https://www.amazon.com/dp/B01NH7OXGV/
http://www.thirumandiram.net/

568 ஏறுதல் பூரகம் ஈரெட்டு வாமத்தால் ஆறுதல்
கும்பம் அறுபத்து நாலதில் ஊறுதல் முப்பத் திரண்டதி ரேசகம் மாறுதல்
ஒன்றின்fகண் வஞ்சக மாமே
கும்பகம்

568 Ēṟutal pūrakam īreṭṭu vāmattāl āṟutal
kumpam aṟupattu nālatil ūṟutal muppat tiraṇṭati
rēcakam māṟutal oṉṟiṉfkaṇ vañcaka māmē
kumpakam

568
Purakam is defined as
INHALATION from LEFT Nostril
For matra six and ten

Kumbhakam is understood as
RETENTION
For matra four and sixty

Rechakam is defined as
EXHALATION from RIGHT Nostril
For matra two and thirty

This is called Pranayama.

If done the other way (inhalation through right nostril and exhalation through left nostril) it may cause damage. So always INHALE from LEFT, EXHALE from RIGHT, with RETENTION for both inner and outer breath.

Hatha Yoga Pradipika

https://www.amazon.in/dp/8185787387
https://www.ashtangayoga.info/philosophy/source-texts-and-mantra/hatha-pradipika/
https://www.sanskrit-trikashaivism.com/en/hatha-yoga-pradipika-asana-pure-translation/623

अत्याहारः प्रयासश्च प्रजल्पो नियमाग्रहः ।

जनसङ्गश्च लौल्यं च षड–भिर् योगो विनश्यति ॥१.१५॥

atyāhāraḥ prayāsaśca prajalpo niyamāgrahaḥ ।

janasaṅgaśca laulyaṃ ca ṣaḍbhir yogo vinaśyati ॥ 1.15 ॥

1.15
Too much and too many food-items swallowing
Over work of humungous, long, tiring hours
Chatter and gossip, being too talkative and gullible
Becoming fanatic in rules, regimes, and blind vows

Promiscuous, keeping mixed company, submissive in body
And
Lacking in Trust, Discipline or Conduct, being of wavering mindset

These are the 6 great obstacles and blocks on the Path of YOGA.

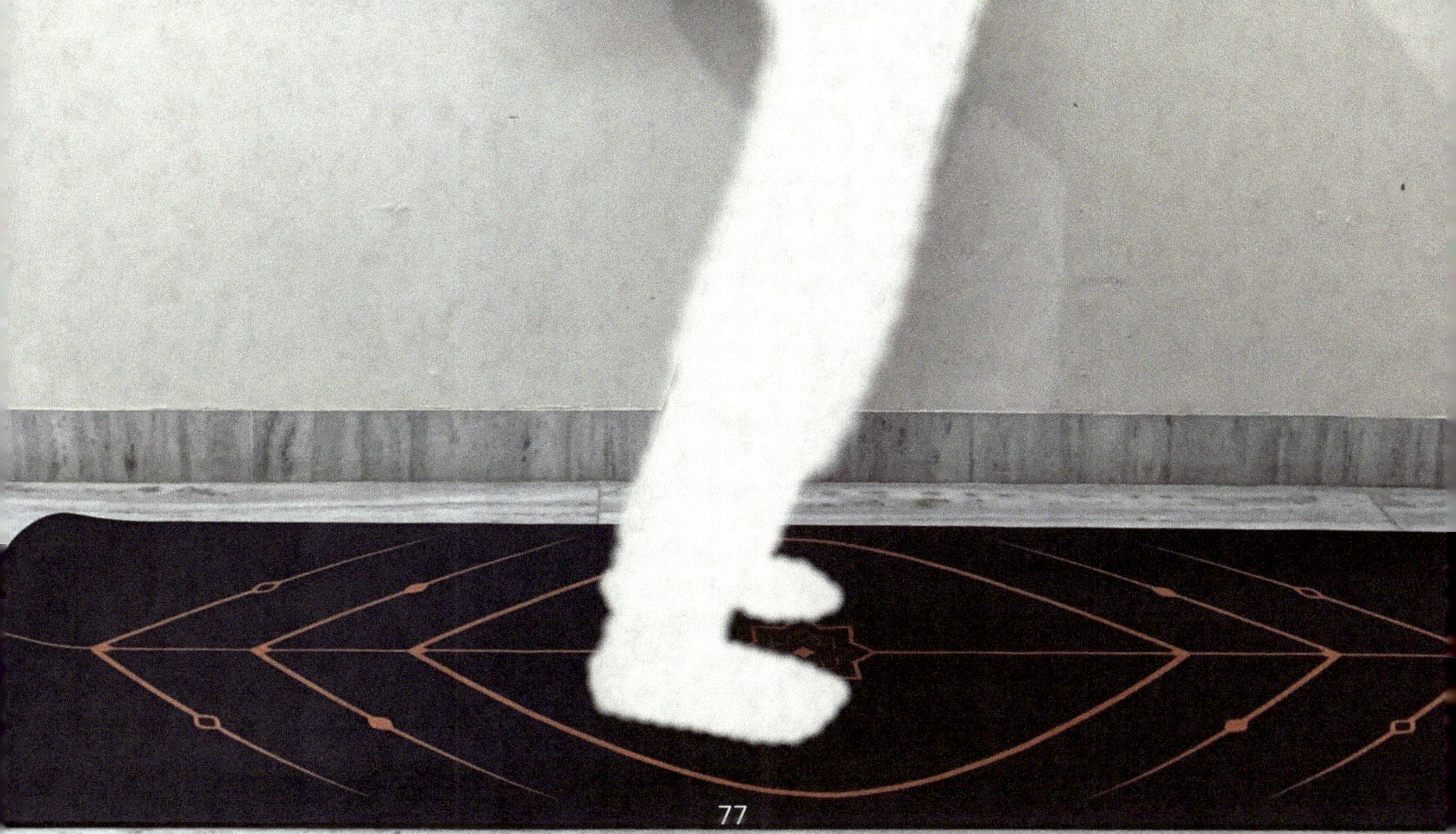

Gheranda Samhita

https://en.wikipedia.org/wiki/Gheranda_Samhita
https://www.exoticindiaart.com/book/details/gherand-samhita-HAA136/

उपविश्य आसने योगी पद्मासनं समाचरेत् । गुर्वादि–न्यासनं कुर्याद् यथैव गुरुभाषितम् ।

नाडीशुद्धिं प्रकुर्वीत प्राणायाम–विशुद्धेये ॥ ५.३८

5.38 Being well seated, the Yogi, in Padmasana pose,
Having first remembered various deities, and following the Guru's teaching in cheerful earnest,
Nadi Shodhana Pranayama is begun for cleansing the Nerves and subtle energy Channels.

वायुबीजं ततो ध्यात्वा धूम्रवर्णं सतेजसम् । चन्द्रेण पूरयेद्वायुं बीजं षोडशकैः सुधीः ॥ ५.३९ ॥ चतुःषष्ठ्या मात्रया च कुम्भकेनैव धारयेत् । द्वात्रिंशन्मात्रया वायुं सूर्यनाड्या च रेचयेत् ॥ ५.४० ॥ उत्थाप्याग्निं नाभिमूलात् ध्यायेत् तेजोऽवनीयुतम् । वह्निबीजषोडशेन सूर्यनाड्या च पूरयेत् ॥ ५.४१ ॥ चतुःषष्ठ्या मात्रया च कुम्भकेनैव धारयेत् । द्वात्रिंशन्मात्रया वायुं शशिनाड्या च रेचयेत् ॥ ५.४२

5.39 Chandra nadi = Ida nadi = left nostril inhalation for 16 counts. 5.40 Then 64 counts of holding the breath within. Then exhalation from Surya nadi = Pingala nadi = right nostril for 32 counts.
5.41 Again inhalation from right nostril for 16 counts,
5.42 Then retention within for 64 counts and exhalation from left nostril for 32 counts.

NOTE – In modern Nadi Shodhana, we do not hold the breath. Secondly we are not worried about the counts. We simply do alternate nostril breathing with awareness and silent soft breath, without breath retention. This is very purifying and less taxing, hence doable by one and all.

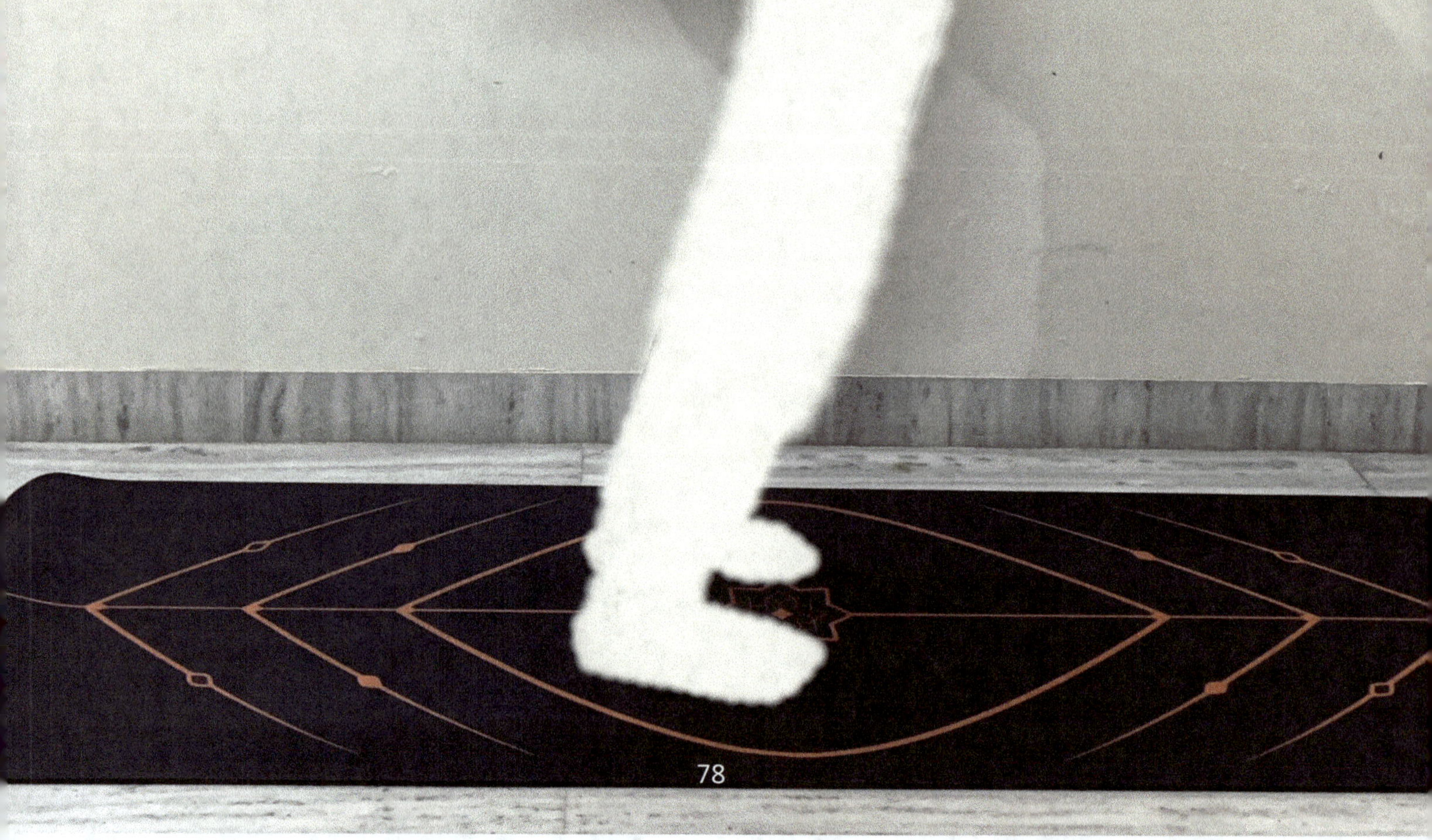

Surya Namaskars For Health, Efficiency & Longevity

The first available treatise on asana sequence that has become famous as Surya Namaskar. Published in book form in 1929 by Bhawanrav Shrinivasrav Pant Pratinidhi, the Rajasaheb of Aundh.

http://www.suryanamaskarforworldpeace.org/history.html
https://www.amazon.in/Surya-Namaskars-Ancient-Indian-Exercise-ebook/dp/B0827Y35WT

Suggested Reading

Asana Pranayama Mudra Bandha
The standard text on Yoga practice by Swami Satyananda Saraswati, Bihar School of Yoga.
https://www.biharyoga.net/asana-and-pranayama.php
https://www.amazon.com/Asana-Pranayama-Bandha-Fourth-Revised/dp/8186336141/

Research paper on Yoga by Himika Sharma
https://pubmed.ncbi.nlm.nih.gov/31181300/

Iyengar Yoga
https://www.iyengaryoga.in/bks-iyengar

Krishnamacharya Yoga Mandiram
https://www.kym.org/

Sri Sri School of Yoga
https://srisrischoolofyoga.org/in/

Ashwini Kumar Aggarwal
– Patanjali Yoga Sutras – 1st – 2018 – Devotees of Sri Sri Ravi Shankar Ashram, Punjab.
– Bhagavad Gita Applied Wisdom – 1st – 2018 – Devotees of Sri Sri Ravi Shankar Ashram, Punjab.
– Prashna Upanishad – 1st – 2020 – Devotees of Sri Sri Ravi Shankar Ashram, Punjab.

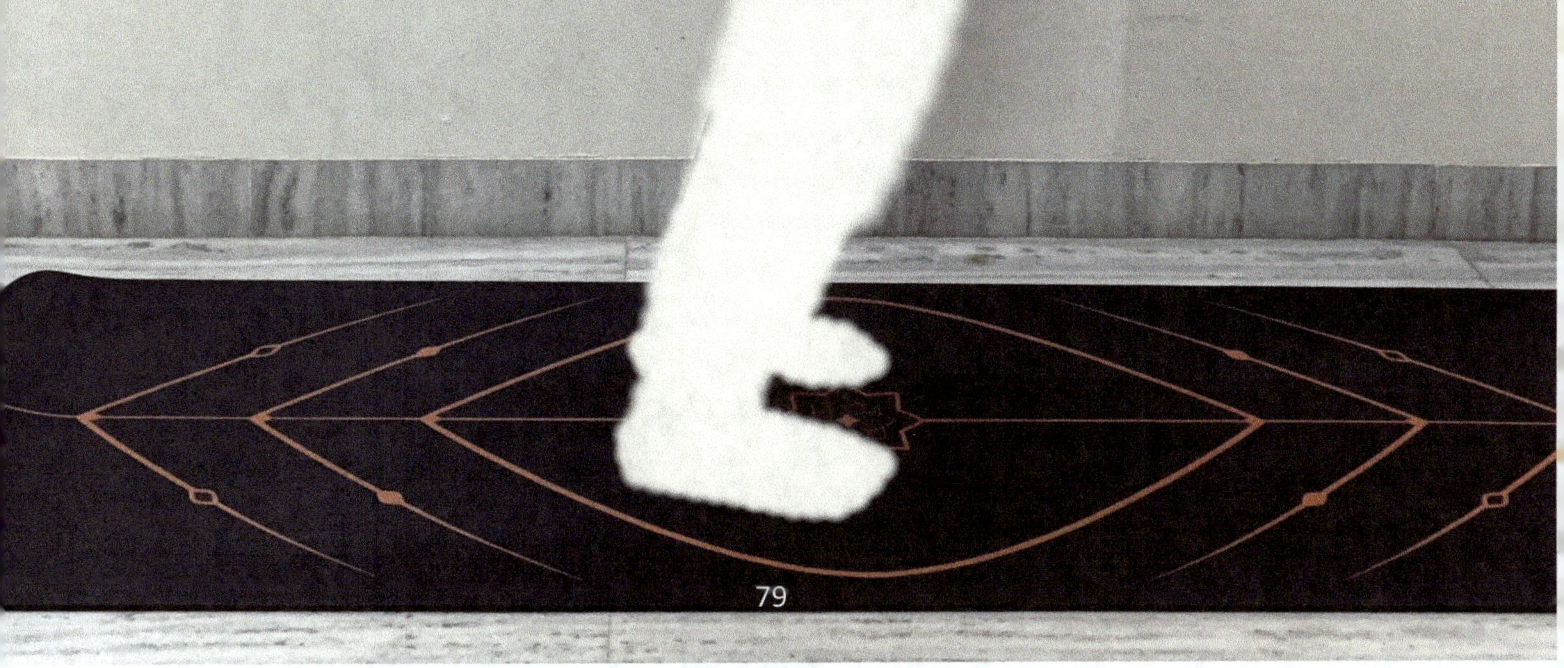

Epilogue

When one stops still and listens, Consciousness is heard. Felt.
The nature of Consciousness is to expand, blossom, shine and share. Yoganidra and Meditation easily make it heard. Yogasana and Pranayama awaken its delight, and life becomes Blissful.

सर्वे भवन्तु सुखिनः । सर्वे सन्तु निरामयाः ।

सर्वे भद्राणि पश्यन्तु । मा कश्चिद् दुःख भाग् भवेत् ॥

ॐ शान्तिः शान्तिः शान्तिः ॥

When faith has blossomed in life,
Every step is led by the Divine.

Sri Sri Ravi Shankar

Om Namah Shivaya

जय गुरुदेव

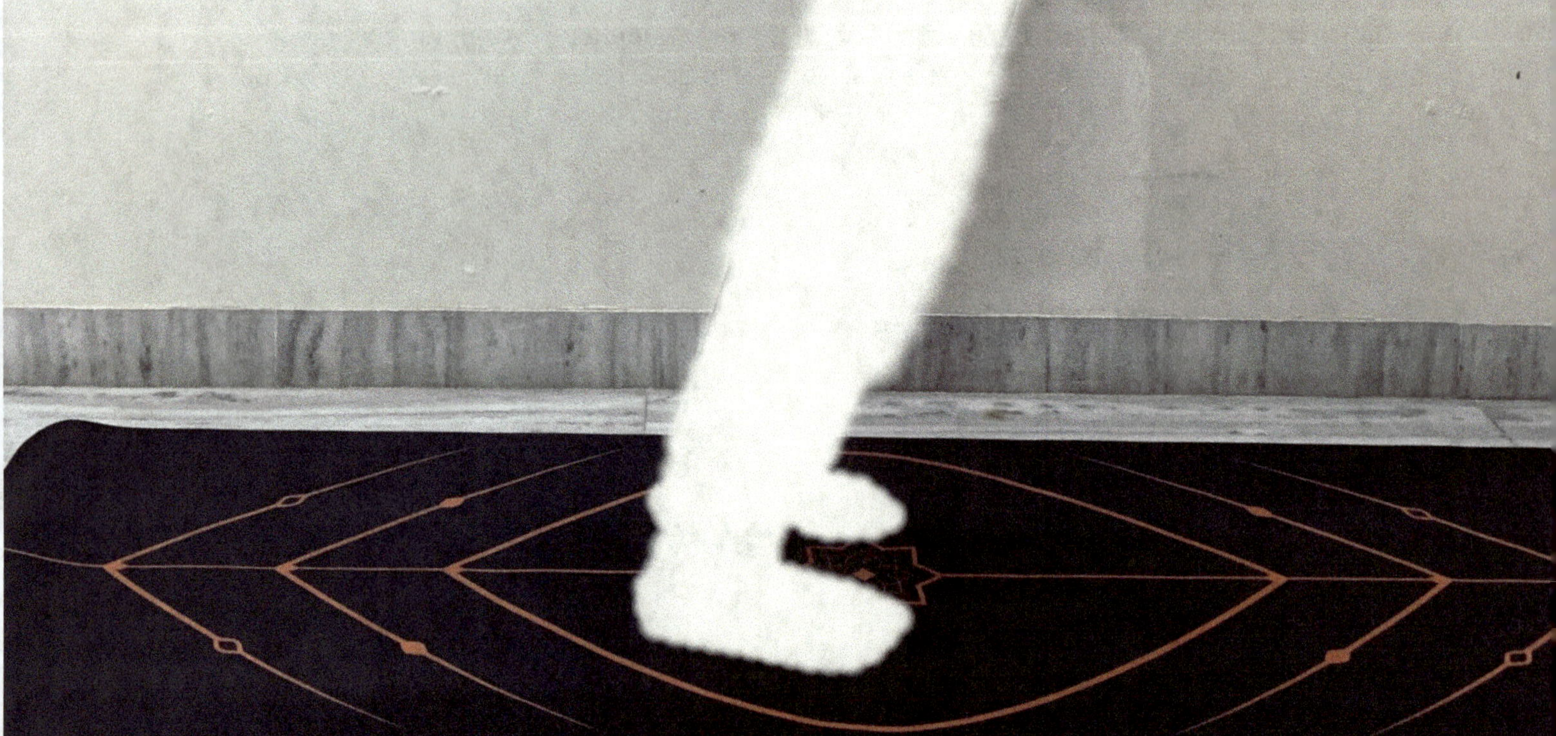

www.ingramcontent.com/pod-product-compliance
Lightning Source LLC
LaVergne TN
LVHW082232080526
838199LV00107B/365
* 9 7 8 9 3 9 5 7 6 6 4 2 5 *